Trans and Non-binary Gender Healthcare for Psychiatrists, Psychologists, and Other Health Professionals

This is an expert, focused and authoritative clinical overview of trans health care. Barrett and Richards combine many, many years' experience in the field, and reach out wisely, not only to psychiatrists and psychologists but to multi gender specialist professions in shaping affirmative and collaborative care with the trans and non-binary people we serve.

Matthew Mills, Consultant Speech and Language Therapist Tavistock and Portman NHS Foundation Trust; President of the British Association of Gender Identity Specialists (BAGIS).

Christina Richards and James Barrett have produced an authoritative yet accessible book on the range of issues involved in Trans and Non-binary gender healthcare. For too long different health care professions have felt siloed, practicing from within different stand-alone contexts, aware that their practice was limited by the specificity of their discipline. This book illustrates the importance of thinking broadly about the medical, psychological, religious, relational and psychiatric dimensions of healthcare and how these can usefully inform each other. It puts trustworthy, up to date knowledge into the hands of a range of practitioners. By bringing such disparate bodies of knowledge together our ability to serve our gender diverse clients with sensitivity and competence is significantly extended. A real aid to holistic thinking and practice that can only be a major resource for practitioners from different disciplines.

Professor Martin Milton, Regent's University London, UK.

Both Professor Christina Richards, an Applied Psychologist and Dr James Barrett, a Consultant Psychiatrist have written a comprehensive guide for other health care professionals working with trans and non binary people. This book covers a wide range of topics that is educational but also accessible. Both clinicians are widely respected in the health care for trans and non binary people and have extensive experience in this field. They have written a book that is hugely helpful for a better understanding and learning about trans and non binary people. It is an engaging book and provides you with valuable information that will help you to see the complicated political, social, cultural and health barriers that many trans and non binary people experience when trying to get adequate care. An excellent book, long overdue.

Dr Kamilla Kamaruddin, GP in East London, RCGP Inspire Award 2019.

Trans and Non-binary Gender Healthcare for Psychiatrists, Psychologists, and Other Health Professionals

Professor Christina Richards
Charing Cross Gender Identity Clinic and Regents University London

Dr James Barrett
Charing Cross Gender Identity Clinic

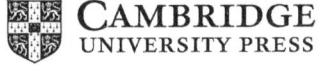
CAMBRIDGE
UNIVERSITY PRESS

CAMBRIDGE
UNIVERSITY PRESS

University Printing House, Cambridge CB2 8BS, United Kingdom

One Liberty Plaza, 20th Floor, New York, NY 10006, USA

477 Williamstown Road, Port Melbourne, VIC 3207, Australia

314–321, 3rd Floor, Plot 3, Splendor Forum, Jasola District Centre,
New Delhi – 110025, India

79 Anson Road, #06–04/06, Singapore 079906

Cambridge University Press is part of the University of Cambridge.

It furthers the University's mission by disseminating knowledge in the pursuit of
education, learning, and research at the highest international levels of excellence.

www.cambridge.org
Information on this title: www.cambridge.org/9781108703024
DOI: 10.1017/9781108628419

© Christina Richards and James Barrett 2021

First published 2021

A catalogue record for this publication is available from the British Library.

ISBN 978-1-108-70302-4 Paperback

....

Every effort has been made in preparing this book to provide accurate and up-to-date information that is in
accord with accepted standards and practice at the time of publication. All case histories are amalgams and do
not represent any one individual, living or dead. Nevertheless, the authors, editors, and publishers can make
no warranties that the information contained herein is totally free from error, not least because clinical
standards are constantly changing through research and regulation. The authors, editors, and publishers
therefore disclaim all liability for direct or consequential damages resulting from the use of material
contained in this book. Readers are strongly advised to pay careful attention to current national and
international guidelines, as well as information provided by the manufacturer of any drugs or equipment
that they plan to use.

Contents

Acknowledgements

Christina's Acknowledgements

I would first like to thank my co-author Dr James Barrett FRCPsych for his knowledge, wisdom, and friendship since I was a dumb kid with a fair bit to think with, but yet not much to think on. It saddens me that far too few people see his tireless work 'behind the scenes' advocating on behalf of gender diverse people to colleagues who would doubtless never listen to a lesser clinician, but who almost inevitably do to him – and so change their practice for the better in response to his penetrating and always compassionately moral arguments. For very many trans and non-binary people, his hand has removed obstacles without their awareness. This is as it should be, but it is also certainly worth recording here.

I would also like to thank all the trans and non-binary people I have seen over the years for sharing their experiences – both joyous and saddening – with me, and so providing a depth of knowledge and wisdom of which a book such as this can merely scratch the surface.

This book is, of course, also dedicated to Phil – words can never say enough, though I write a hundred books and fill them all with a single acknowledgement to you. I would also like to thank Professor Martin Milton for believing in me, more than once and when it really counted, and for inspiring me to be kind as well as clever – and to use clever to be kind. To Frances, Carlo, and all of the managerial and administrative staff who work so hard to make everything happen and, it seems, never get the credit they deserve. To Drs Seal, Berner, and Nambiar for their invaluable technical advice and to Dr Sally Hodges for being smart and compassionate and for steel in approximately equal amounts – and all to the end of helping others. To my mother who modelled how one can change the system from within, and to all the activists I have had the pleasure of meeting who have modelled how to change it from without. To Rio for becoming more impressive every day, and for allowing me to be constantly delighted and surprised by the direction that takes. To Margie for completing the crosswords I cannot get with grace, and then being a most wonderful friend as the years pass. For Chris for letting me share land and time (and whiskey) with him. And for Frances (I must have been an – ahem – 'interesting challenge' – which you managed with never less than grace).

Lastly this book is dedicated in memoriam to Dinah, "The best little cat in the world". She really was.

James's Acknowledgements

My thanks, of course, to the thousands of patients it has been my privilege to try to help over the past thirty-two years. They have taught me everything I know. My colleagues at the Charing Cross Gender Identity Clinic need to be thanked for helping me work out what it all means and most particularly Christina Richards, who additionally provided the encouragement, nagging, cajoling, and hounding (as appropriate) that helped get this book into print; I hope she forgives me having done exactly the same to her.

Finally, and most importantly, my thanks to lovely Sally who bravely kept our show on the road when I should have been pulling my weight and was instead sequestered away with a laptop.

Author Biographies

Professor Dr Christina Richards BSc (Hons), MSc, DCPsych, CPsychol, EuroPsy, FBPsS is an HCPC Registered Doctor of Applied Psychology and a full Fellow of the British Psychological Society (BPS), where she is the current Chair of the Division of Counselling Psychology; committee member for Psychologist Prescribing; Lead National Assessor for Counselling Psychology; Chair of the revision committee of the *BPS Diagnosis – Policy and Guidance*; and Chair of the revision committee of the *BPS Guidelines for working therapeutically with sexual, gender, and relationship diverse clients,* of which she was an original co author.

Professor Richards is Visiting Full Professor of Gender and Mental Health at Regent's University London School of Psychotherapy and Psychology. She is Lead Consultant Psychologist/Head of Psychology at the London Gender Identity Clinic (Charing Cross) within the Tavistock and Portman NHS Foundation Trust. This role involves strategic planning and management on a national and international level, supervising senior staff, assessing people with highly complex needs for hormones and surgeries, and supervision of individual and group therapies from a number of different modalities.

Professor Richards is also Head of Research at the NHS London Gender Identity Clinic (Charing Cross) within the Tavistock and Portman NHS Foundation Trust. This role involves responsibility for the strategy and implementation of the research programme at the clinic. Professor Richards also lectures and publishes internationally on gender, sexualities, and critical mental health both within clinical academia and also to third-sector and statutory bodies.

Professor Richards was elected to the Executive Board of the European Professional Association for Transgender Health (EPATH) and was selected by the Executive Board of the World Professional Association for Transgender Health (WPATH) to be lead chapter author for Adult Assessment in the *Standards of Care Version 8* (SoC v8) revision. She also represented the East Midlands to NHS England's Clinical Reference Group (CRG) on Gender Identity Services and is listed as an expert in gender diversity by the BPS on the Gender Diversity Specialist Register (whose criteria she co-drafted). She is one of the few psychologists recognised by HM Courts and Tribunals Service as a specialist in the field of gender dysphoria, thus allowing her to prepare medical reports for the Gender Recognition Panel.

Professor Richards is a founding member of the British Association of Gender Identity Specialists (BAGIS), a past trustee of the National LGBT Foundation, a founding member of BiUK, and co-author of the *Bisexuality Report*.

Professor Richards is Editor-in-Chief of the journal of the British Psychological Society's Division of Counselling Psychology: *Counselling Psychology Review*. Her own publications consist of various papers, reports, and book chapters. She is first author of a clinical guidebook on sexuality and gender published by Sage: *Sexuality and gender for mental health professionals: A practical guide* (2013); first editor of the *Palgrave handbook of the psychology of sexuality and gender* (2015); first editor of a multidisciplinary book about people who identify outside the gender binary of male or female: *Genderqueer and non binary genders* (2018); and sole author of the monograph *Trans and sexuality – An existentially informed ethical enquiry with implications for counselling psychology* (2017).

Dr James Barrett MB, BS, BSc, MSc, FRCPsych is Director of the Tavistock and Portman Charing Cross Gender Identity Clinic. He has worked at the clinic for thirty-two years, as Director since 1999. He sat on the intercollegiate working party that drew up the UK Standards of Care for people with Gender Dysphoria, sat on the NHS England Clinical Reference Group, and is a founding member and the elected first President of the British Association of Gender Identity Specialists (BAGIS).

He is editor of and major contributor to the first textbook aimed at working clinicians and has advised and informed the policies of the Human Fertilisation and Embryology Authority, the UK penal estate, the Civil Service, and many large corporate organisations.

Dr Barrett has lectured and broadcast on this subject, nationally and internationally, in more places than it is sensible to list.

Introduction to Gender Diversity

Introduction

People who are not content to remain the gender they were assigned at birth have existed throughout human history and in all recorded cultures (Herdt, 1996). Naturally the experiences of people in the contemporary high-income cultures which are the focus of this book will be informed by the understandings and technology available now, but fundamentally gender diversity is not a new phenomenon. It is therefore curious that, until recently, it was commonly thought that gender diversity was so rare that it would not trouble most psychiatrists or psychologists in their usual course of work. This is no longer the case, as there has recently been an exponential increase in the number of gender diverse people coming forward, which mirrors that of same-sex-attracted people a couple of decades before. Most likely this is once again due to the greater, although still tenuous, social acceptance being shown towards sexual and gender diversity in some countries. It follows therefore that psychiatrists and others will have seen gender diverse people throughout their careers, but without necessarily being aware that they were doing so. Indeed it was not uncommon for the authors – both senior National Health Service (NHS) Consultants in Gender Identity Healthcare – to have seen gender diverse people who were excoriating about the care they had received in mainstream mental health services, only to reply upon asking that they had not told the clinicians there about their gender issues – an omission which makes good-quality care almost impossible as we shall see later in this book. Gender forms a key part of the people we see and, while not necessarily being the focus of the work, naturally informs how we go about it.

It is not uncommon therefore for the community or inpatient psychiatrist or psychologist to be faced with a gender diverse patient and to feel the need to *do the right thing* but not be quite sure what that thing might be. Does one manage the gender? The presenting mental illness? Both? What about the feelings of staff? Other patients? Which ward does one accommodate the patient on? What, when we get right down to it, does one call them? Fear not. The answers to these very reasonable questions are happily rather more simple than one might fear and are contained within the very book you now hold in your hands.

We should note here that this is a clinical book intended for use in clinical settings. If you are after elaborate academic arguments, abstruse wording, or dozens of citations on each point, then this is not the book for you. The book is indeed based in the academic literature, although for readability we have not usually cited it in detail. The lists of further reading at the end of each chapter will give a useful direction for citations in each area, as will the occasional citations throughout the text. The content of this book also rests, as so much of this field does at present, on the expert opinion of the authors and our colleagues. With the basis of the work outlined then, let us turn first of all to the different sorts of folk one might meet and go from there.

In contemporary high-GDP cultures, trans and non-binary people can broadly be categorised into the following four groups:

1. **Binary trans people.**This includes people who were assigned male at birth and who identify as (are) women where one should use *Ms, Mrs, Miss* and *she, her,* and so on. It also includes people who were assigned female at birth and who identify as (are) men where one should use *Mr* and *he, his,* and so on.

2. **Non-binary people with a fixed gender identity.**This includes people who identify as other than strictly male or female and who have a fixed gender. For example, on a notional gender spectrum from male to female, one might identify as roughly 60% male or as 70% female. Many non-binary people prefer the use of *Mx* as a title and to be referred to as singular *they*, although some may wish to use *he* or *she* according to their predominant gender identity.

3. **Non-binary people with a fluid gender identity.**Again, this group of people identify as other than strictly male or female but in this instance have a fluid gender which varies according to circumstance or individual feelings. As earlier, many in this group prefer the use of *Mx* and to be referred to as singular *they*, although again, some may wish to use *he* or *she* according to their predominant gender identity at that time.

4. **Agender people.**Agender people have no gender.[1] Note that having no gender is not the same as having aspects of both genders.[2] Similar to non-binary people, agender people often prefer the use of *Mx* and to be referred to as singular *they*.

Other terms include *eunuch* for people who identify outside the traditional notions of masculinity or femininity (and is more common for people assigned male at birth) and who wish to have their genitalia removed, but not necessarily other interventions. Separately, *genderqueer* people also take umbrage with the very notion of a gender binary.

While we have listed the most commonly used terms here, a great many others are in use and vary according to the current thinking in the communities or derive from other cultures. The terms here are the safest bet at the time of writing, but it is always best to ask the patient what their preferred terms are and to use those.[3] We should also note that some patients use reclaimed terms such as *queer* or *tranny* which may be preferable to that specific patient but are highly offensive to others. It should not be assumed that because a term is safe to use with one patient, it will be so for all. In this book we will generally use *trans* to refer to both [binary] trans people and non-binary people, but we will also occasionally use *gender diversity* as these are the safe(st) terms at the time of writing. We will also use the term *cisgender* (the antonym to trans) to refer to those people who are content to remain in the gender they were assigned at birth.

There can be the question of how to refer to people in the usual sorts of forms one invariably has to fill out as a patient in healthcare settings. A balance must be struck between having usable data and not excluding or offending people. Although not specifically recording agender people, the British Association for Sexual Health and HIV (BASHH,

---

[1] Sometimes these people are also known as Neutrois people.
[2] Liking both Victoria sponge and chocolate cake is not the same as disliking both.
[3] And you can, of course, always blame us for any disliked terms contained in this book and so maintain rapport.

2019) has the following eminently sensible suggestion to address this issue, which is formed of two interlinked questions:

Q1 Gender identity – Which of the following options best describes how you think of yourself?
  ○ Female (including trans woman)
  ○ Male (including trans man)
  ○ Non-binary
  ○ In another way*
  ○ Not stated (person asked but declined to provide a response)
  ○ Not known (not recorded)
  * Coded as "Other" in the NHS data dictionary
Q2 Is your gender identity the same as the sex you were assigned at birth?
  ○ Yes
  ○ No
  ○ Not stated (person asked but declined to provide a response)
  ○ Not known (not recorded)

Many of the various terms discussed earlier rest on a notion of a gender binary of male or female; however, the difficulty with this expressed by genderqueer people is not as unreasonable as one might, at first, expect. Physiological intersex conditions of all sorts occur at 1.728% in the general population (Blackless et al., 2000), a rate which does not consider neurological intersex – although we are thinking in this book largely of gender (psychological and social) rather than biological sex. Even in gender, however, people have far more similarities than differences. There are in fact *no* differences of kind between male and female psychology, with those few differences of degree having a vastly larger overlap than difference (in statistical parlance, there may occasionally be a statistically significant result but always with a tiny effect size).

The differences we see are therefore more to do with culture than specific underlying factors. Perhaps this is because gender is not actually a linear spectrum which would necessitate an increase in masculinity being perfectly inversely correlated with a decrease in femininity – the genders are not 'opposite'. Let us consider risk taking, for example. We might consider that to be a 'masculine' trait and expect it to be more prevalent in males than females – but what do we mean by risk taking? How about a woman who wishes to have a baby in conditions of extreme deprivation? This instance poses a significant risk of death to both mother and child, yet we tautologically discount such risk from [gendered] risk taking on the basis that it is traditionally a feminine activity. We might similarly consider aggression which in nature is naturally at its most severe in females protecting young. It becomes difficult to bottom out on what we mean by masculinity and femininity – and on what underpins them.

And yet people *do* have some sense of their gender; it is just difficult to point to what that is and where it comes from. Perhaps the best metaphor would be that of language. We know that there is a genetic predisposition towards language, but not a specific language. Genes are needed to code for neurological and physical development in order to speak, with the type of language determined by culture and the way the language is expressed by the individual being determined by psychological factors, social situation, and education. A complex interplay of genes, psychological and personal environment, and social environment allows, encourages, and discourages certain traits from evolving. To say that this is 'nature or nurture' is to misunderstand the complex interaction of both.

So too is this the case with gender, where genes and personal and social development all interact to create something which feels 'natural', but which is in fact the result of the interplay of many factors. Indeed, a good deal of work suggests that at least some trans people have a genetic predisposition and that the in utero differentiation of the brain and the genitals in different trimesters may be a reason for trans people having brains (and genders) which are at odds with their genitals (and so birth-assigned sex). A good deal of evidence suggests that some trans people have brain regions in line with their gender of identity, but not birth-assigned sex (e.g. Bevan, 2015), which also gives a simple reason why trans identities persist in the face of such significant social opprobrium, and indeed unethical aversion and conversion 'therapies' which invariably fail (see Chapter 5, *Supporting Trans and Non-binary People in Mental Health Services*). Naturally the personal expression of all of this in the social sphere is determined by cultural factors.

Note here we are using *assigned at birth* to refer to the gender which is assigned when a baby is delivered and inferred from an inspection of their genitals. Thus we may have a person who was *assigned male at birth* (AMAB) or *assigned female at birth* (AFAB), which are the preferred terms when we need to refer to the sex and gender someone was assigned at birth.[4] We don't use 'natal male' or 'natal female' or 'male to female' ('MtF') or 'female to male' ('FtM') anymore because these terms imply that the trans person 'was' of their birth assigned gender and then changed; which was not the experience for many trans people. Certainly a gender was assigned and often reinforced (sometimes coercively) until such time as the individual was in a position to express themselves – but it was never actually their felt or internally experienced gender. Thus to refer to assignation of gender at birth is reasonable, to refer to *being* that gender at birth is not. Note also that referring in this way is *only* done when it is absolutely necessary to refer to the gender assigned at birth – which is very seldom. As with any other congenital condition which has little impact on adult day-to-day functioning, such as a closed atrial septal defect, we do not continually define the person by it or continually refer to it. Instead we absolutely do acknowledge it only in those situations where it is relevant and not elsewhere – at surgery for the person with the septal defect or upon an endocrine consultation for a trans person. Otherwise trans people should be referred to as their gender of identity – trans men (AFAB) are simply men, and trans women (AMAB) are simply women.

Diagnosis and Formulation

While trans people are not defined by being trans and indeed generally spend their lives doing the ordinary sorts of things one might expect such as working, studying, having families, paying taxes, poking their phones, and so on, there are some occasions in the clinical setting where being trans is relevant, and where an appropriate diagnosis may be necessary. Diagnosis, including the various options available as well as correct formulations, are considered thoroughly in Chapter 2, *Assessment*; suffice to say here that trans is not a mental disorder (WHO, 2019), although higher rates of anxiety and depression can occur

---

[4] It's rank sophistry to say that only sex, and not gender, is assigned at birth. The genital inspection and following sex assignment immediately lead to a set of cultural practices which constitute gender. Indeed, some hospitals go so far (and so soon) as to have pink or blue scissors to cut the umbilical cord.

if the person is subject to abuse, stigma, prejudice, or discrimination, or is unsupported in their gender (see Chapter 5, *Supporting Trans and Non-binary People in Mental Health Services*). Instead, trans is best considered simply as something like pregnancy or sexual expression which is a part of the human condition and may require medical or psychological assistance. Indeed, while this book includes a good deal on trans and non-binary people who have had, or who are seeking, treatment such as hormones and surgeries, it is important to recognise that trans people are very much more than that; many trans and non-binary people identify and present in a variety of ways without seeking any medical or psychological attention at all. Thus the work of diagnosis and formulation consists of identifying any differentials and situating the person's gender within their wider life.

A medical doctor or increasingly an applied psychologist (the usual types being counselling psychologists or clinical psychologists in the United Kingdom (UK)) may make the diagnoses and formulation associated with gender diversity due to the biological-psychological-social approach considered central to this work and the central place of psychology in this field. This work by medical doctors or applied psychologists includes recommendations for hormones or surgeries, although naturally any prescribing or surgery will need to be carried out by clinicians specialising in prescribing or surgery.

While gender diversity is not usually very complex, it can be so, and clinicians must be competent to recognise differentials (WPATH, 2011). It is therefore quite unacceptable to 'have a go' without sufficient knowledge and experience. For this reason, the Royal College of Physicians (RCP) in the United Kingdom is currently leading on a post-qualification masters-level course in gender identity healthcare, which is also open to applied psychologists; the British Association of Gender Identity Specialists (BAGIS) has strict entry criteria for full membership (BAGIS.co.uk). This is not to say that generalist clinicians or specialists in other fields cannot see trans people for the areas they specialise in, but that they should be cautious about trans-related diagnosis and should not initiate specialist gender treatments without having been trained by people who are already expert in the field.

Continuing professional development (CPD) is also most important for those who see trans people in any setting, as this is such a fast-moving field. Unless one is a gender specialist, there is no need for in-depth specialist knowledge; however, there is a need for a basic level of knowledge such that one is culturally competent, as it were. As a rule, one should have the level of basic knowledge needed for another group – thus, if one is aware of hormone replacement therapy for cisgender women, one should be for trans women too (Richards & Barker, 2013). There may well be a point in both cases at which one refers to an endocrinologist, but to profess *no* knowledge is clearly unacceptable. We should point out that gaining that knowledge from (potentially stressed) patients is not acceptable – that is properly the place of (paid) CPD and many clinicians and community groups will be very happy to provide it.

That mention of community groups is important also, as much good information can be found both there and in the grey [community] literature. Indeed, it can be useful for clinicians who are seeing many trans clients, and who are not engaging with the communities already, to do so. Naturally if one is not a community member,[5] one should not invade semi-private community space or groups; however, an arranged visit or enjoying an open

---

[5] It is always important to bear in mind that many medical doctors and psychologists are also trans.

Pride event can be both fun and useful as it avoids the pitfalls of the *clinician illusion*.[6] It can also be useful to become comfortable using words associated with gender and sexuality, perhaps especially community terms. For example, we need to know and be able to use terms such as *packer*[7] and *binder*[8] and to be able to say the word "fuck", because if our patients use them we also need to. If our patient confides, that; "I'm worried I won't be able to fuck my partner", we may need to reply, "In what way are you worried about not being able to fuck your partner?" If we say "In what way are you worried about … ahem … making love … with your partner?" the patient is unlikely to give a forthright response. It can be useful to practise saying out loud any terms such as *fuck* one feels uncomfortable with.[9] It can feel a bit silly at first but does pay dividends in patient rapport and history taking.

Children and Young People

In this book we are primarily concerned with people older than the age of majority, which in the United Kingdom is age 18. This group is considered, in the usual course of things, to necessarily be independently capacitous and therefore able to make decisions about their own care. Of course this does not mean they can instruct a clinician to act in a certain way, as the clinician must either agree with the proposal or set out a range of possible proposals for a discussion with the patient about their preferred option. In all cases the clinician is ultimately responsible for providing care which they believe is in the patient's best interest. There are, of course, 18-year-olds going on 25 who are measured and considerate and with whom one may have a very adult to adult conversation. There are also 18-year-olds going on 14 who are still in a very adolescent stage of development and who require careful management, especially with regards to permanent physical changes.[10]

That said, at present, the very few people who do express regret about their gender-related decisions tend not to be young people but rather people in their very late 20s to early 50s who have a sexualised approach to gender diversity and who make physical changes (most often obtained in the private sector and very often abroad) predicated on their sexuality rather than on a more quotidian basis (see Chapter 8, *Sexuality, Relationships, and Reproduction* for more on this sort of issue). Younger people, if they have regrets, tend to be concerned with *how* they did it, rather than *that* they did it; thus, it can be useful to encourage people to study or work in addition to transitioning, rather than just focusing on the transition – such that they have both an occupation and an appropriate gender, rather than just a gender when they are done with transition. Naturally, discussion of reproductive options is vital for this group and is considered in Chapter 8, *Sexuality, Relationships, and Reproduction*.

---

[6] For those unfamiliar with this term, it applies when a clinician who only sees a set of people through their clinical work is consequently only able to see them through a clinical lens. The psychiatrist who only sees trans people at work may consider all trans people to have some form of psychopathology – because 100% of the people they have [knowingly] met have indeed been mentally ill. But *of course* they have. Were they to go to dinner with some trans people without mental illnesses, they would have another view and the illusion would be broken.

[7] A prothesis used to give a masculine genital contour.

[8] A tight elastic undershirt used to flatten one's chest.

[9] Although perhaps not while on a bus or while attending a Parent Teacher Association meeting.

[10] The flounce into the consulting room while looking at their phone with the eye-roll and exhalation at any undesired utterance by the clinician being pathognomonic for this.

Some may think that young people are too young to know what their gender is, but a moment's consideration reveals this to be fallacious. After all, we do not question whether cisgender people know what their gender is at a young age. Of course, we must be cautious about significant physical interventions in case the young person evolves with a different consideration of gender as they develop. However, the longer the young person has held their conviction, the more likely it is to carry on through adolescence and adulthood. A staged approach whereby a person is allowed to express and explore their gender from a young age, with support and education for those around them, with puberty-blocking medication giving a little more thinking time at a later stage, followed by cross-sex hormones and then surgeries in late adolescence or early adulthood after years of gender dysphoria would seem reasonable and indeed has proved very successful.

Note also that 'watchful waiting' (or "doing nothing" as some trans people would term it) is not neutral – to go through such a crucial period in one's life as adolescence in the wrong gender, unable to interact appropriately with one's peers, can be the cause of very significant psychological and social damage. Whether acting or not acting, there is no 'neutral' option.

We should note here that for both young people and adults, discomfort with their gender is not necessarily the same as expressing their gender. While decisions about significant physical interventions will often be predicated upon an expressed change of gender, as it is important to see if a person is able to function in their gender role, there may have been discomfort about their gender beforehand which the person did not feel able to express. Young people with the most unsupportive parents may be the most likely to hide their gender. Indeed their parents' lack of support predicated upon the fact that there had not been prior expression of gender diversity may in fact simply be evidence of the reason the trans person felt unable to be out in the first place.

In all cases, a measured approach is needed, which respects the young person's expression and development and links pragmatics to aspirations – just as with all other areas of young people's development.

Intersectionality

When considering gender diversity, age is just one area which inflects how we might work with clients. Many other demographics will inflect how a person perceives themselves, as well as how they perceive us, including ethnicity, (dis)ability, religion, class, income, and so on. These elements are considered throughout this book; suffice to say here that they inflect gender and also one another. A wealthy, white, middle-class trans woman with no disabilities will have a very different experience from someone who shares none of those things except her gender. It is imperative that psychiatrists and psychologists consider people in a holistic manner and avoid diagnostic overshadowing where trans becomes the sole defining feature of the person. It may be pertinent; it may not be at all; but it is, in all cases, only one aspect of the person in front of us.

Current Guidance

This book is written by two of the most experienced clinicians in transgender care globally and draws on the latest research, community sources, and many years practising in the field. It also takes into account many of the guidelines and resources which are available to clinicians; many of them are included in the Further Reading section at the end of the chapter. As this book is published by the Royal College of Psychiatrists in the United Kingdom, these include the Royal College of Psychiatrists' 2013 *CR181: Good practice guidelines for the assessment and treatment of adults with gender dysphoria*; and the 2018 *PS02/18: Supporting transgender and gender-diverse people*; the British Psychological Society's 2019 *Guidelines for psychologists working with gender, sexuality and relationship diversity*. Further, we have also drawn upon the authors' other books in this field which have global applicability, and we encourage you to read them.[11] In 2016 the United Kingdom's Royal College of Nursing produced *Fair care for trans patients: An RCN guide for nursing and health care professionals* which may also be profitably read. The American Psychiatric Association's *Diagnostic and statistical manual* (DSM) and the worldwide *International statistical classification of diseases and related health problems* (ICD) diagnostic classifications are considered in Chapter 2, *Assessment*; we also draw your attention to the eighth edition of the World Professional Association for Transgender Health's (WPATH). *Standards of Care*, which should be published in 2020. In the meantime, the 2011 seventh edition is extant. Lastly, the Yogyakarta Principles are extremely useful for those with an interest in human rights.

With all these references, and indeed with other clinical guides and the academic literatures, we caution that this is a fast-moving field, with constantly evolving cultural and subcultural understandings. This means that information quickly becomes out of date, with ten years probably the maximum time one can have a good degree of faith in any sort of publication. Indeed, when it comes to the legal and policy details, events can move rather faster than that. Thus when considering a course of action, certainly refer to authoritative guides such as this and those mentioned earlier but also consider the clinical situation and the most compassionate way we may assist the person in our consulting room at that time.

Cultures and Subcultures

The person one sees in the consulting room will almost certainly have a cultural background and may have a culturally derived understanding of gender – not least because trans people have been found globally in all cultures and all times. It is beyond the scope of this book to give a comprehensive account of the history and ethnography of gender diverse people, but as a background we shall content ourselves with a brief, and necessarily insufficient overview.

As stated at the start of the chapter, trans people have been found from America across Europe and Asia to Polynesia (Herdt, 1996), and from the Bronze Age across recorded history to the present day. Of course a Bronze Age understanding will not match that of a person living in contemporary London or New York, and indeed options differ between London and New York – just as cisgender expression varies across time and geographical/cultural regions; however, the fundamental notion of people with one body living in the way culturally expected of the other is ubiquitous. In the modern world, people in New Zealand or Australia have options to select the 'X' category on their passport rather than 'M' for male or 'F' for female and so have options available which people in London or New York do not have. Similarly income, (dis)ability, and other factors will determine what options one may have in different cultures.

---

[11] Beautifully written and very reasonably priced.

In America the First Nation peoples have 'two-spirit' individuals who are often people assigned male at birth who take on aspects and roles of femininity or people assigned female at birth who take on aspects and roles of masculinity, but they do not always take on all of the aspects or roles of the 'other' sex. Two-spirit people traditionally have a healing or spiritual role as a medicine person (in the First Nation sense of the word) or as a nurse, although this will by no means always be so, with two-spirit people holding a variety of roles according to their wishes, ability, and cultural standing.

The First Nation peoples use several terms for two-spirit people according to tribal background. These include *hwame* by the Mohave, *nádleehé* by the Navajo, *wíŋkte* by the Lakota, and *ilhamana* by the Zuni, in addition to others. These terms are not precisely analogous and, in common with many cultural terms, defy direct translation into English – a most important point for readers based in a two-gender and two-sex cultural system. Indeed, *two-spirit* itself is not a term which is universally or uncritically accepted, as it suggests a system of understanding which does not accord with all First Nation understandings.

The Samoan *fa'afāfine* (lit: the way of a woman) people are in some ways similar to two-spirit people, although naturally different in other ways and within a specific cultural context which inflects basic understandings about the world. Fa'afāfine people are usually assigned male at birth and engage in traditionally feminine behaviours and are often particularly community oriented. Within Polynesia, there are also other gender diverse peoples such as the *fakaletī* of Tonga who are assigned male at birth and have a female identity, and the *māhū* from Hawaii and Tahiti who are assigned male at birth and have female gender identities and are attracted to men.

In India, the *Hijra* people may identify as men, [trans] women, or as third gender; in 2014, their status as a third gender was legally recognised. Hijra are traditionally assigned male at birth, are devotees of the Bahuchara Mata, and may officiate at some Hindu ceremonies. Hijra often gain their spiritual power through removal of their genitals and through living as women, not uncommonly in all-Hijra communities, both for fellowship and due to discrimination. However, as with many gender diverse cultures, some people identify as Hijra outside this strict definition. Some who in the past might have identified as Hijra now use the term *khwaaja sira* instead of Hijra and may identify with the [Western] notion of gender incongruence.

Sadly, many of the cultural terms previously detailed have been adapted into vernacular slang as terms of abuse, perhaps because many cultures which had previously embraced gender diversity have grown less tolerant as a result of the evangelisation of native peoples during historic colonisation and more recently with the spread of other restrictive under-standings through cultural colonialism. This marginalisation of gender diverse people has led some to seek legal recognition, as with the Hijra, and others to adopt the medical discourse from post-industrial nations, instead of the traditional understandings touched on earlier. This can lead to increasing isolation for gender diverse people as communities no longer have a place for gender diversity, which in turn can lead to minority stress, home-lessness, and work in underground economies where further exploitation can occur. However, the rise of the identities of trans, transgender, and genderqueer within some cultures, while supplanting traditional understandings, can offer community or a sense of identity to gender diverse people who would otherwise be marginalised.

As well as global and historic cultures, gender diversity has a number of other cultural aspects. These include religious views, which we have included in Chapter 9, *Legal and Religious Aspects*, given the edicts on gender which accompany most religious scripture. In addition, BDSM (bondage and discipline, dominance and submission, and sadomasochism), as well as fetishism have some cultural understandings and practices related to gender and are considered in Chapter 8, *Sexuality, Relationships, and Reproduction*. It remains for us here to consider a couple of subcultures which relate to gender but do not fit wholly under any of the previously discussed cultures or subcultures – *cosplay, furries, and Bronies*.

Cosplay

The interests and identities discussed next can seem unusual or even alarming to those unfamiliar with them, but we would urge the reader who has not had experience of them to exercise caution in any assumptions, as these identities are, fundamentally, harmless and often form fulfilling parts of the lives of those involved. Cosplay is an old phenomenon, perhaps dating to the early years of the past century. The word is a crude translation of a Japanese portmanteau phrase incorporating *costume* and *play* – those who practise are therefore *cosplayers*. They wear costumes (usually self-created and often extremely skilfully done) representing, typically, comic book, video, film, or other notable fictional characters, not uncommonly from anime, although not invariably so. The intention is usually to physically demonstrate liking of, admiration for, or affinity with the character concerned. Abstract concepts or groups, such as football teams, are not the object of cosplaying.

Minor degrees of cosplay are exceedingly common (the wearing of a named football shirt replicating that worn by a favourite named player would be an example) and sometimes more extensive cosplay isn't recognised as such by those who engage in it. One thinks of the large numbers of individuals who attended singalongs of *The Sound of Music* dressed in nuns' costumes or the happy hordes who attend *The Rocky Horror Show* dressed as Frank N Furter or, if less adventurous, Brad or Janet. Large numbers of people enjoy role-playing Roundhead or Cavalier troops and generals as part of the Sealed Knot historic battle re-enactment club. Simultaneously, oddly, as caregivers the same individuals can still express mystification and mild anxiety when their children dress as Japanese cartoon characters and attend comic conventions.

Having made a really superb costume, cosplayers' temptation to show off to others is entirely understandable, and they are to be found at comic book conventions and gatherings of fans of such entertainment franchises as Harry Potter, anime, and Marvel or DC comics. An element of judging each other's costumes is inevitable, and special credit is generally given for particularly detailed costumes which have involved a large amount of personal effort. Cosplayers sometimes formally "compete" in open competition before judges; in these circumstances, they may briefly strike poses characteristic of the character they portray or sometimes perform very short "in character" routines.

Trans cosplay, sometimes termed *crossplaying*, is both common and uncritically accepted in cosplay circles. A cosplayer assigned male at birth who has made a particular effort to emulate a female character will be judged only on the verisimilitude of the costume. No adverse judgement appears to be made on account of bodily incompatibility, possibly because this is the one thing the cosplayer cannot change. Further, a change of sex is not uncommon in Japanese manga and anime in any case, and very often the male characters in such cartoons have a rather elfin, feminine form.

Of interest is that there is a noticeable association between cosplay, autistic spectrum conditions (ASC – see Chapter 7, *Autistic Spectrum Conditions and Intellectual Disability*, for more on this) and gender dysphoria best represented, perhaps, as a Venn diagram with some degree of overlap among the elements. However we should make clear that these behaviours are also commonly undertaken by neurotypical people and may profitably be considered with this group in mind. That cosplaying should attract some people with ASC is not surprising. People with ASC tend to have an intense and detailed interest in their enthusiasms and are often also highly proficient users of the internet. Intense integration with a fandom (this word itself being a portmanteau of *fan kingdom*) often follows and along with it a sea of merchandised products. Only a few further steps are needed before self-manufacture of costumes and an entirely understandable desire to display the skill deployed becomes inevitable. The cosplay coordinator at HyperJapan 2014 in London estimated 10% to 20% of the cosplayers as being on the ASC spectrum.

For people with ASC and gender dysphoria, cosplaying is particularly attractive because it offers an entirely safe space in which to assume a gender identity other than that assigned at birth. Other cosplayers are almost certain to judge femininity or masculinity solely on the basis of what the person can control and manufacture rather than on the bodily constitution that they were born into. The same cosplay coordinator thought that around 5% of cosplayers had some degree of gender diversity.

Strikingly, despite many of the female animation characters portrayed by cosplaying having a decidedly sexualised appearance, cosplaying itself is not sexual. Sexualised behaviour of any sort other than that normally portrayed by the character or sexualised comments by observers – particularly other cosplayers – is uncommon and, indeed, should it occur, is frowned upon.

Furries

Furries are a group superficially similar to cosplayers but, on closer examination, are rather different. Furries are individuals who report feeling an affinity with an animal, often a mammal and frequently a dog, wolf, cat, or bear. There are, of course, global cultural traditions of animal affiliation and identity (see Richards & Barker, 2013). Within contemporary Western cultures, as well as mammals, furries may feel an affinity with a fantastical animal such as a dragon or a unicorn. Whatever the affinity, detailed costumes in keeping with the animal concerned are constructed and worn, and there are similar conventions of like-minded individuals. Cosplayers are often concerned about not being confused with furries.[12] One gets the impression that some view the more common sexual behaviour of furries with suspicion and confusion.

Furries may also feel an affinity with animals of a different sex than that of their birth-assigned [human] gender, and this can be a start, or part, of gender exploration for the person concerned.

Bronies

A Brony is an adult male, usually younger than age 50, with an intense interest in the television series *My Little Pony: Friendship Is Magic*. A much smaller number of females, sometimes termed *Pegasisters*, are involved. Bronies number in the hundreds of thousands and are found throughout the English-speaking countries. Their interest is intense and

---

[12] As one notable cultural commentator indicated: "I don't know why they all have a go at furries? If you want to dress up as a giant rabbit and have relations with a man squirrel that's none of my business. I've seen stranger things. I've *done* stranger things" (Elemental, 2014).

again there is some overlap with ASC. In common with people with ASC, Bronies' interest is not uncommonly raised in settings where it seems inappropriate or boring to others. Although suspected by others of having an inappropriate sexual interest in the little girls for whom the television series was originally intended, such interest seems uncommon and certainly not usually present in those Bronies who have ASC. Again, only a few trans folk seem to come from a Brony background, with those that do tending to identify with the female ponies and as Pegasisters.

It is notable that cosplaying, particularly cross-sex cosplaying, and to a lesser extent furry and Brony affinity, is often an antecedent to an openly expressed distress about assigned gender role and a subsequent change of that role. When one is an independent adult, these things usually are simply a somewhat unusual part of gender exploration. However when a patient is not independent, for example, if they have marked ASC, then to parents or carers it can seem that the change of gender role has, somehow, been 'caused' by the earlier cosplaying or, alternatively, that the expression of gender dysphoria is as light-hearted and superficial as cosplaying is to those cosplayers who don't have gender dysphoria or indeed ASC. In fact, the earlier cosplaying may well have held a deeper, often covert significance for the gender dysphoric cosplayer – enabling the person to experience acceptance in another gender role, albeit in very time-constrained and circumscribed circumstances, much as Halloween parties can be used for this purpose in other settings.

Of course, there can be a temptation to elide cosplay, furries, and Bronies with gender diversity. The (rather trite) idea being that if one can identify as another sex, one can identify as anything else one may wish to be – a wolf, an anime character, or whatever. This argument, while superficially attractive, is spurious – there is a great deal of cross-over between human men and women – including brain and genital differentiation in utero, through childhood, and at puberty – and this is thought to be the basis for much gender identification (Bevan, 2015). In contrast, there is essentially no cross-over between humans and wolves, except at the most basic of levels – and of course none between humans and anime characters. One may have an affinity with wolves or anime, of course, but one is not – essentially – those things. In contrast, the reality of being trans is a fundamental feeling – immovable with 'therapy' or other 'treatments' and with an aetiology backed up by solid science that one is, in a very real sense, another gender.

Summary

In summation, the golden rule of seeing trans people in a clinical setting is to be polite and not to fret or overthink. If in doubt, it can be helpful to substitute another demographic one is more familiar with. For example, if people complain they did not wish to share a ward with a person of a certain ethnicity who was acting wholly appropriately, it can be useful to consider how you would respond in that situation. Responding in the same way for trans people is usually sensible. Once one gets past the feeling of discombobulation that becoming familiar with gender diversity can sometimes provoke, it becomes clear that kindness, politeness, and ethical practice in the best interests of the patient work just as well here as in all other areas of medicine and psychology. While we may occasionally have to make decisions which our patients dislike, if we try to be collaborative and are always respectful and as accommodating as we can be, we will have discharged our duty as clinicians, and indeed as human beings.

Further Reading

American Psychiatric Association (APA). (2013). Gender dysphoria. *Diagnostic and statistical manual of mental disorders 5.* Washington, DC: American Psychiatric Association.

British Psychological Society. (2019). *Guidelines for psychologists working with gender, sexuality and relationship diversity* (2nd ed.). Leicester: British Psychological Society.

(forthcoming 2021). *Guidelines for assessment, formulation, and diagnosis* (2nd ed.). Leicester: British Psychological Society.

das Nair, R., & Butler, C. (2012). *Intersectionality, sexuality and psychological therapies: Working with lesbian, gay and bisexual diversity.* Oxford: Wiley-Blackwell.

Richards, C., & Barker. M. (2013). *Sexuality and gender for mental health professionals: A practical guide.* London: Sage.

Richards, C., Bouman, W, P., & Barker, M. J. (eds.). (2018). *Genderqueer and non-binary genders.* London: Palgrave-Macmillan.

Royal College of Nursing. (2016). *Fair care for trans patients: An RCN guide for nursing and health care professionals.* London Royal College of Nursing.

Royal College of Psychiatrists. (2013). *CR181: Good practice guidelines for the assessment and treatment of adults with gender dysphoria.* London: Royal College of Psychiatrists.

(2018). *PS02/18: Supporting transgender and gender-diverse people.* London: Royal College of Psychiatrists.

World Health Organization. (2019). HA60 Gender incongruence of adolescence or adulthood. In *WHO international statistical classification of diseases and related health problems 11.* Geneva: WHO.

World Professional Association for Transgender Health (WPATH). (forthcoming 2020). *Standards of care* (8th ed.). Minneapolis, MN: WPATH.

British Association of Gender Identity Specialists (BAGIS) – BAGIS.co.uk

European Professional Association for Transgender Health (WPATH) – EPATH.eu

International Lesbian Gay Bisexual Trans and Intersex Association (ILGA) – ILGA.org

World Professional Association for Transgender Health (WPATH) – WPATH.org

Yogyakarta Principles – yogyakartaprinciples.org

References

Bevan, T. H. (2015). *The psychobiology of transsexualism and transgenderism.* Oxford: Praeger.

Blackless, M., Charuvastra, A., Derryck, A., Fausto-Sterling, A., Lauzanne, K., & Lee, E. (2000). How sexually dimorphic are we? Review and synthesis. *American Journal of Human Biology, 12,* 151–166.

British Association for Sexual Health and HIV (BASHH). (2019). *Recommendations for integrated sexual health services for trans, including non-binary, people.* Cheshire: BASHH.

Elemental, P. (2014). Enter the convention: Crespo's Comicon remix. [Recorded by P. Alborough] On *The Giddy Limit* [Digital download]. Brighton: Tea Sea Records.

Herdt, G. (1996). *Third sex, third gender.* New York: Zone Books.

Richards, C., & Barker. M. (2013). *Sexuality and gender for mental health professionals: A practical guide.* London: Sage.

World Health Organization. (2019). *ICD11: Classifying disease to map the way we live and die.* Retrieved 16 May 2019 from: www.who.int/health-topics/international-classification-of-diseases

World Professional Association for Transgender Health (WPATH). (2011). *Standards of Care for the health of transsexual, transgender and gender nonconforming people* (7th ed). Minneapolis MN: WPATH.

Assessment

Introduction

Assessment of trans and non-binary people falls broadly into two forms: the usual assessment carried out in mental health services for mental health concerns which is somewhat adapted to accommodate trans patients or specialised assessment for hormones and surgeries which is usually carried out in National Health Service (NHS) gender identity clinics. While many readers will be unlikely to carry out the latter, we have also included details of that assessment here. After some general introductory remarks, we shall take these two forms of assessment in turn; note also that this consideration of general assessment may usefully be read alongside Chapter 4, *Mental Health Conditions*.

Assessment, whether for purposes of diagnosis, formulation, or both, usually seeks to collaboratively establish the nature of the client's distress and often to situate it within their wider life. This will require an appropriate general history which focuses on the pertinent matters of the presenting condition but does not ignore elements such as sexuality, relationships, and gender which may not apparently be related but may nonetheless prove useful in determining the best way of helping the patient (BPS, forthcoming 2021).

For trans people, there will naturally be some consideration of gender, but this should not overshadow other elements of the person's life. Clinicians must be careful not to miss important facts by focusing on gender unduly. We might imagine, for example, an assessment of a trans person where childhood abuse is missed because the clinician is focusing on childhood gender atypicality – an egregious error which would lead to much poorer treatment outcomes. Similarly, in formulation we should be careful not to over-attribute to gender. Suggesting that the gender atypicality is a result of childhood abuse misses the fact that gender atypical children are often targeted by abusers precisely because they are socially isolated due to being gender atypical – the abuse follows the gender atypicality rather than vice versa. A balanced, nuanced approach to assessment of trans people is vital.

Do also bear in mind that trans people who have been in contact with mental health services may be wearied by constant assessment or exploration of their gender.[1] Very often systems are set up such that repeated assessment is required – but in order to establish rapport, undue questioning should be minimised through referring to notes and/or disregarding questions unrelated to the presenting concern. As always, prurient interest must not drive questions. It is, for example, extremely rare that one needs to know the genital status of a patient. Asking "have you had the operation yet?" is extremely intrusive and

---

[1] This is happily abating somewhat for same-sex-attracted people, but there was a period where this was pursued ad nauseam to no particular end within the psy- professions. Hopefully understanding of the assessment of gender atypicality will progress similarly.

usually unnecessary and demonstrates ignorance of the fact that many trans people do not have [genital] surgeries.

We must also be careful of assuming that questions relating to gender should always be aimed at trans people. Trans people may well have thoroughly explored their gender as part of being trans. In contrast, cisgender people have usually not explicitly considered the implications of their gender, assuming it is 'natural' or 'normal' if they have considered it at all. However, we know that a number of conditions are related to unconsidered gender norms – such as anorexia in young cisgender women (and increasingly men), steroid abuse in young cisgender men, high rates of completed suicide in cisgender men who feel bound by expectations of masculinity not to express emotion, and so on. In such instances, gentle exploration of gender with cisgender patients may be of more benefit than excessive focus on the gender of trans people.

General Assessment of Trans People

The basis of any successful assessment is rapport. Naturally if there is no rapport, or if the patient is actively hostile, an effective assessment cannot be made. It follows therefore that respecting the gender of the patient is a necessary requirement of effective assessment. Unless there is an extremely strong reason to think otherwise – such as florid psychosis in a person with no history whatsoever of gender dysphoria – preferred names and pronouns should be used. This should not be predicated on legal change, as some people are too chaotic to engage in bureaucratic and costly changes of gender – but should instead be based on their stated preferences. If one is unsure, it is entirely reasonable to discreetly ask. There are occasions in the clinical setting when legal name and gender must be recorded in such instances, recording legal name and gender, while using the patient's preferred name, title, and so on elsewhere is recommended (see Chapter 5, *Supporting Trans and Non-binary People in Mental Health Services* for more on single-sex accommodation).

Aside from the good manners of using the patient's preferred name and pronouns, it should be borne in mind that trans and non-binary people have not been well served by psychiatrists and psychologists in the past. This includes the historic use of shock and emetic 'therapies', behavioural interventions, and conversion 'therapies' to try to stop people from being trans. Indeed, unfortunately some psychiatrists and psychologists still consider trans and non-binary people to necessarily be mentally ill (they are not – WHO, 2019a). It follows therefore that some trans and non-binary people are understandably wary and indeed some may be actively hostile. As far as possible, do try not to take this personally, for we are at the start of a style of practice which is more accommodating of diversity – and some might argue that in our field it is not before time. We can mitigate this a little before people sit down with us. Simple things such as a small rainbow flag on the front door, a diversity of magazines and pictures in the waiting room, patient demographic forms and questionnaires which have non-binary options (and do not list white, male, heterosexual, and married at the top of each list), and reception staff who do not misgender patients[2] will all pay dividends.

Once in the assessment, the usual questions will apply, but do bear in mind that some elements may need adaptation – if assessing or using psychometrics, one cannot use

---

[2] Using the first letter of the first name and the surname (e.g. "J Doe") for all patients can be good practice here as it does not specify gender.

birth-assigned sex as a baseline because trans patients will necessarily not follow population norm behaviours or cognitions for that sex. Unfortunately, population norms for the gender of identity (there are none for non-binary people) will not usually work either, as socialisation in the birth-assigned gender will affect these. Inferential tests such as the Rorschach test are not valid as the inferences cannot be made on this population without spurious theorising (see Chapter 10, *Psychotherapy*). In all cases, a robust clinical assessment which takes into account the specific nature of the patient is vital.

As stated earlier, when conducting the clinical interview, it is vital not to be over-concerned about trans to the exclusion of the matter under consideration. As a rule, it is better to have trans as a *possible* inflection, rather than a go-to cause. The idea of a 'whisper over one's shoulder' as to whether this particular issue might be to do with the person being trans, rather than a neon sign over the patient's head saying "↓ *TRANS!* ↓", can be a helpful one. Let us consider a short vignette:

> *Karen is a trans patient who is depressed because she had a break-up after ten years of relationship. With some exploration, you find that the break-up was precipitated by her having had an affair, which itself was caused by the relationship becoming 'stale'. She tells you she is saddened by the thought that her partner was the person who supported her through transition years ago; and so she feels especially guilty.[3]*

We can see here how Karen being trans *inflects*, but does not *cause*, the depression. Further, we can see how an undue focus on Karen being trans, and [incorrect] assumptions about that, might lead to the supposition that the depression could be something to do with surgeries or hormones, that the partner is the one who had an affair, that the affair was because Karen is trans, and so on. Not only would following any of those assessment 'paths' have been incorrect, but many would have damaged rapport.

If one usually asks medical questions, then it is quite reasonable to ask about hormones or surgeries as part of the usual questions about medicines and surgeries, but it is helpful to establish rapport first and to clearly signpost that this is about medicines and surgeries in general, rather than hormones or trans surgeries specifically. As ever, there must be a reason for the questions and so unnecessarily intrusive questions should be avoided. It should be borne in mind that very often trans people would rather not have had to have had hormones and surgeries and would like to simply get on with life in their gender. For this reason, some may not recount their hormones, surgeries, or gender in full, or indeed at all, even when asked directly. Much reassurance may be needed as to the purpose of the information sought – and couching this in a medical, mechanistic way (drug interactions, etc.) can be useful as it makes apparent that this is not about the person's gender per se but more about the chemical processes in their body at any one time. Having said that, when gaining information about medicines, it is important to ask about hormones (see Chapter 3, *Physical Treatments for Trans People and Their Interactions with Psychiatric Treatments*) and so efforts should be made in that regard.

As a side note, we should mention that clinicians undertaking physical assessment and medicine administration should, in general, not be the same as those undertaking the psychiatric assessment – not least because many trans people have an abuse history and recounting such a history to someone who then physically inspects you can be re-traumatising.

A few other adaptations are necessary specifically for trans people. A general consideration of the effects of marginalisation can be useful – although again this will not inevitably be

---

[3] Karen is an amalgam, and not a real person.

so; substance misuse and risky behaviours may be important to explore if there are other forms of vulnerability alongside; a consideration of undiagnosed autistic spectrum conditions and therefore misattributed behaviours as well as social/work/educational needs is often useful (see Chapter 7, *Autistic Spectrum Conditions and Intellectual Disability*). Lastly, do bear in mind that trans and non-binary people may have been ostracised by their families or have left work or family because they (wrongly) believe that they will necessarily be ostracised. When recording or drawing a genogram, do give due consideration to family of choice[4] which may be composed of friends and partner(s).

Specialist Assessment of Trans People for Hormones and Surgeries

The Arguments for and against Assessment

At the moment, trans and non-binary people who wish to have cross-sex hormones or gender-related surgeries in the United Kingdom must have an assessment by a medical doctor or a statutorily regulated counselling psychologist or clinical psychologist. This differs somewhat globally, with recommendations in the World Professional Association for Transgender Health's (WPATH) *Standards of Care Version 7 and 8* (WPATH 2011, forthcoming 2021). Do bear in mind that these global standards are necessarily reflective of the varying health provisions available globally.

In nationalised healthcare systems such as the United Kingdom's National Health Service, it would seem reasonable to have a high standard of assessment and assistance. While each clinician will naturally adapt to the patient, and somewhat to their own style, the key documents to provide guidance for medical doctors and applied psychologists undertaking such assessments are the WPATH *Standards of Care*; and; guidance from the British Association of Gender Identity Specialists (BAGIS); and the British Psychological Society's Guidelines for *assessment, formulation, and diagnosis* (BPS, forthcoming 2021). Readers should be cautioned, however, that the WPATH guidance has global applicability and is therefore not written with a sole country's medical-legal situation and health economy in mind; and some guidelines are becoming dated in such a fast-paced field.

Entirely legitimate questions are being asked about whether there is a need for assessment of trans people at all. [Psychiatric] assessment made sense under the old theory that trans and non-binary identities are psychopathological – with physical interventions simply being a (somewhat extraordinary) treatment for mental disorder, reluctantly prescribed due to the failure of other forms of intervention such as aversion 'therapies', psychotropic medication, and psychodynamic conversion 'therapies'.

With the contemporary understanding that gender diversity is simply a part of natural human diversity and is not a mental disorder (WHO, 2019a), there is a question as to whether an approach which is simply facilitative of patient requests should be employed in the absence of assessment. This is one version of the Informed Consent model[5] which, at its

---

[4] Sometimes called a *framily*.
[5] Unfortunately there is no strict definition of this model, which makes the debates surrounding it correspondingly fraught with misunderstanding and ill feeling.

hardest end, eschews even physical assessment – with risk being solely within the purview of the patient. The difficulty with this, of course, is that in most medico-legal contexts, the prescribing doctor or operating surgeon *does* hold responsibility irrespective of the wishes of the patient. This responsibility not only includes physical risk but also psychological or psychiatric risk. Indeed, many of the risks are psychological or psychiatric in nature – for example, is the person psychotic? Is this an autistic special interest? Is this body dysmorphia? (See *Differential Diagnoses or Formulations for Gender Diversity* in this chapter and Chapter 3, *Physical Treatments for Trans People and Their Interactions with Psychiatric Treatments*).

It follows therefore that a prescribing GP, endocrinologist, or surgeon may quite reasonably ask a colleague skilled in identifying such differentials – a psychiatrist or counselling psychologist or clinical psychologist – to assess the patient beforehand. Having a psychologically skilled colleague assess a patient has an added advantage in that many of the difficulties (rather than differentials) that trans people face are psychosocial in nature – for example, difficulties with coming out, relationship issues, sexual issues, and education and employment issues – consequently clinicians skilled in these areas also are well placed to assist.

Whatever one thinks about the risk arguments detailed here (and of course the medico-legal placement of risk varies globally), there is another discussion concerning settings where healthcare is paid for by someone other than the patient – and that is whether there is likely to be benefit from the treatments. In nationalised healthcare, taxpayers have a right to expect that their taxes (which after all they have no choice but to pay) are spent on something which is necessary, rather than just something someone wants. This is why one cannot get a tattoo of a favoured football team paid for by the United Kingdom's National Health Service – there may be no harm, the patient may consent and indeed desire it, but there is no likely medical benefit either. Of course, the patient is entirely at liberty to spend their own money on it but cannot compel the taxation of a classroom assistant, for example, to be spent on their tattoo just because they very much want it. In healthcare economies which are free at the point of provision, therefore, only certain procedures are available[6] and clinicians are charged in determining not only whether they are safe but also whether they are likely to actually benefit the patient.

In all this, there is a balance, of course, between a draconian assessment process which excludes any 'false positives' (i.e. people who are not trans) but causes significant distress to trans people who must be so assessed over a very significant period of time; against a hard Informed Consent model which has no distress caused by assessment but allows the most vulnerable (those who are still developing, have significant mental illness, have an autistic special interest, have some forms of fetishism, etc.) to make irreversible mistakes on the basis that these are their mistakes to make. This latter is a sort of very right-wing 'devil take the

---

[6] There is another debate about what should be available. That hormones as well as chest and genital/reproductive surgeries are available is entirely reasonable given the huge benefits these provide to well-assessed patients. Additionally, if one wishes to be crass about it, the improvement causes a substantial financial saving in terms of mental health services and substantial additional income taxes as mentally healthy trans persons are able to earn more. On that basis, it is reasonable to argue for facial surgeries and proper hair removal to be available from the NHS.

There is sometimes an argument that these things are not freely available to cisgender people; however, the benefits are proportionally greater for trans people who have fewer cues as to their gender and are thus less able to engage in society without these treatments – with the concomitant disability this causes.

hindmost approach' of course. The balance, as ever, is somewhere in between – with the least necessary assessment which still protects the most vulnerable. In some sense, this is not a matter for clinicians as the medico-legal aspects are a matter for the law and regulators. Until statutorily regulated clinicians have their responsibility abrogated, some form of assessment will always be needed. We should note here too that it is not possible for patients to sign for, or otherwise abrogate, that responsibility – the assessing clinician is always responsible and therefore cannot be compelled to act in a way which they, personally, believe not to be in the best interests of the patient – irrespective of any other consideration. Similarly, until the NHS or other healthcare economies are willing to pay for what patients want – rather than what clinicians agree they need – there will need to be some form of assessment. The question therefore naturally turns to what the nature of that assessment might be, given the situation we find ourselves in.

Current Assessment Protocols

Assessment in this field is, in essence, remarkably simple – consisting, as it does, of just six words:

1. Is it trans?
2. Will it work?

Naturally things become more complex when the theory meets reality – but the basis is to determine whether there are any differentials which might better describe the presenting gender diversity (in general, there are not, but we must make sure) and to make a formulation and diagnosis; and then to determine whether the interventions the patient is seeking will benefit them (now). Let us consider these in turn before looking at the sorts of things which would be considered in a standard assessment.

Differential Diagnoses or Formulations for Gender Diversity

Such differential diagnoses are few and rather uncommon. Indeed, in general, psychiatric or psychological practice it would be somewhat unusual for these to be the reason for a person to present with gender diversity – vastly more likely is the fact that the person is indeed trans or non-binary. Nonetheless, these are important considerations, for to give significant physical interventions to people who are not trans would be to do them a grave disservice and cause irreparable harm.

Psychosis

Psychosis is considered in full in Chapter 4, *Mental Health Conditions*, but we shall note here that if the psychosis ebbs and flows along with the gender dysphoria, it is likely that the person is not trans, but that the gender is a facet of the psychotic illness. If, however, the person remains gender dysphoric irrespective of the current remittance of their psychosis, then they are likely to be trans *and* have a psychotic illness.

Body Dysmorphic Disorder

Body dysmorphic disorder (BDD) is similarly considered in full in Chapter 4 *Mental Health Conditions,*. Here we will note that when the BDD is linked to a 'gendered' body part in the absence of a wish to live in a different gender role, it is likely to be BDD. However, if it is in the context of a genuine wish to be of another gender, then it is likely to be simply that the trans person has an understandable wish not to have the wrong body parts for their identity or has become obsessed with that body part in the context of gender dysphoria.

Sexual Fetishism

Sexual fetishism is considered in full in Chapter 8, *Sexuality, Relationships, and Reproduction*, suffice to say here that if the drive to transition is sexual in nature, then upon transition that drive will likely abate through the day-to-day familiarity of the gender role. This can leave the person with neither the sexual enjoyment of cross-gender play nor the drive to transition. Naturally if the drive has gone but permanent changes remain, there can be significant decompensation on the part of the patient.

Secondary Gain

Some people find benefit from changing gender role aside from the comfort afforded by living in the correct gender. The most common of these is secondary gain by offenders who are seeking abrogation of responsibility, more attention, or special treatment (see Chapter 6, *Supporting Trans and Non-binary People in Forensic Settings*); however, there are, of course, also trans offenders who must be differentiated.

Other people seeking secondary gain can be those who feel isolated, marginalised, or socially awkward. People with these difficulties can find spaces, not uncommonly online, where warm, welcoming trans people offer kindness and support not otherwise experienced on the reasonable assumption that anyone in a trans support group is likely to be trans (as indeed they most often are). These isolated people can therefore sometimes convince themselves that they are a part of this group by being trans. There can also be something of a cachet to being trans[7] – to being an interesting person who is not like other people *and for that reason and not due to some personal 'flaw'*. This can be very appealing to some people who have struggled to socially integrate. Conversely, of course, many trans people first find themselves through online exploration and find online support to be invaluable.[8]

ASC Special Interest

This matter is considered in full in Chapter 7; suffice to say here that there is a very high rate of people with autistic spectrum conditions (ASC) who are *also* trans and therefore simply having an autistic spectrum condition is by no means a differential in and of itself. In those rare cases where there is a special interest in the absence of gender dysphoria, the presentation varies such that there is usually little wish to actually live in a different gender role – rather, the interest is far more theoretical and abstract.

Possible Diagnoses and Formulation

Having considered differentials, what possible diagnoses might pertain in the case of gender dysphoria? In considering this, the health taxonomy used locally will naturally be followed; however, these do vary a great deal and we generally recommend the use of the latest edition of the World Health Organization's *International classification of diseases and related health problems* (currently with the 11th edition in implementation form), as this is both the most

---

[7] Although a cachet which can have a high cost in discrimination.

[8] And maybe trans and non-binary people *are* a bit special – certainly a number of cultures globally and historically have thought so (Herdt, 1996).

recent and has a truly global reach. Nevertheless, we shall consider several of the most common next.

Gender Dysphoria

In the American Psychiatric Association's (APA), *Diagnostic and statistical manual* (DSM) of mental disorders – Version 5 (2013), the diagnosis for gender dysphoria is listed as follows:

A. A marked incongruence between one's experienced/expressed gender and assigned gender, of at least 6 months duration, as manifested by at least 2 of the following:

1. A marked incongruence between one's experienced/expressed gender and primary and/or secondary sex characteristics (or, in young adolescents, the anticipated secondary sex characteristics)
2. A strong desire to be rid of one's primary and/or secondary sex characteristics because of a marked incongruence with one's experienced/expressed gender or, in young adolescents, a desire to prevent the development of the anticipated secondary sex characteristics)
3. A strong desire for the primary and/or secondary sex characteristics of the other gender
4. A strong desire to be of the other gender (or some alternative gender different from one's assigned gender)
5. A strong desire to be treated as the other gender (or some alternative gender different from one's assigned gender)
6. A strong conviction that one has the typical feelings and reactions of the other gender (or some alternative gender different from one's assigned gender)

B. The condition is associated with clinically significant distress or impairment in social, occupational, or other important areas of functioning. (APA, 2013a, p. 452)

Note that it refers to " ... the other gender (or some alternative gender different from one's assigned gender)" throughout, thus including non-binary as well as binary genders. It has also been renamed from *Gender Identity Disorder* in the DSM IV to *Gender Dysphoria* in the current DSM 5 in recognition of the fact that it is not a mental disorder (APA, 2013b) and moved from the previous chapter *Sexual and Gender Identity Disorders* in the DSM IV-TR to a chapter all of its own in the DSM 5 to reflect the fact that it does not fit within any other mental health conditions. Indeed, it is worth noting the addition of criterion B to *Gender Dysphoria* in the DSM 5 such that the diagnosis does not apply unless there is " ... clinically significant distress or impairment ... "; gender atypicality alone is insufficient. Sensible clinicians will not elide minority or marginalisation stress here – the distress must be due to being trans, not from being subject to abuse.

Of course, it is somewhat paradoxical to detail a condition which is not a mental disorder in a manual of them; however, the diagnosis was retained in order to ensure funding – especially through insurance schemes in the United States which require a diagnosis for reimbursement. The criterion B therefore becomes contentious as some people do not experience significant distress – perhaps because they are very psychologically robust or are well supported but would still benefit from assistance, perhaps as prophylaxis against just such distress.

Gender Dysphoria has also been used as a sort of proxy in other countries where *F64.0 Transsexualism* from the 1992 ICD 10 has become increasingly anachronistic, although since the recent publication of the ICD 11 including *HA60 Gender Incongruence*, this has become less common.

F64.0 Transsexualism

World Health Organization (WHO) *International classification of diseases* (ICD) – 10th Edition (1992)

Transsexualism is now an obsolete diagnosis which has been superseded by *HA60 Gender Incongruence of adolescence or adulthood* (see later discussion). The former description was:

> A desire to live and be accepted as a member of the opposite sex, usually accompanied by a sense of discomfort with, or inappropriateness of, one's anatomic sex, and a wish to have surgery and hormonal treatment to make one's body as congruend as possible with one's preferred sex. (WHO, 1992).

Note that this refers to a putative 'opposite' sex, implying that men and women are opposite in some way – that the more one is of one, then the less one is of the other – which is understood now not to be the case (see Chapter 1, *Introduction*). This diagnosis therefore does not consider non-binary people in the way contemporary diagnoses do. In addition, the term itself has taken on a little of the inevitable patina medical terms develop over time. Trans people therefore generally do not use 'Transsexual' or 'Transsexualism' and the terms used here of *trans* or *non-binary* are preferred – unless one is making a formal diagnosis, in which case *HA60 Gender Incongruence of adolescence or adulthood* should be used.

HA60 Gender Incongruence of Adolescence or Adulthood

World Health Organization (WHO) *international statistical classification of diseases and related health problems* (ICD) – 11th Edition (2019b) The is as follows:

> Gender Incongruence of Adolescence and Adulthood is characterized by a marked and persistent incongruence between an individual's experienced gender and the assigned sex, which often leads to a desire to 'transition', in order to live and be accepted as a person of the experienced gender, through hormonal treatment, surgery or other health care services to make the individual's body align, as much as desired and to the extent possible, with the experienced gender. The diagnosis cannot be assigned prior the onset of puberty. Gender variant behaviour and preferences alone are not a basis for assigning the diagnosis.
> Exclusions:
> Paraphilic disorders (6D30-6D3Z) (WHO, 2019b)

The ICD has recently been revised and at the time of writing the WHO has released the ICD 11 in its implementation version. In this latest version, *F64.0 Transsexualism* – now rendered obsolete – has been superseded by *HA60 Gender Incongruence*. The diagnosis is no longer classified as a mental disorder and so has been renamed and moved from *V Mental and behavioural disorders/ F64 Gender Identity Disorders/ F64.0 Transsexualism* in the ICD 10 to *17 Conditions related to sexual health/Gender Incongruence/Gender Incongruence of adolescence or adulthood* in the ICD 11.

Note that, similar to *Gender Dysphoria* in the DSM 5, this diagnosis refers to " ... an individual's experienced gender" which takes account of non-binary as well as binary genders. It also makes clear that gender 'variance'[9] alone is insufficient to merit a diagnosis, a measure which is intended to avoid the pathologisation of gender atypical people who do not wish for treatment. As this is the latest, global, diagnosis it is naturally this which we recommend using.

There are other diagnoses which may be considered if those previously given do not pertain – for example, in the ICD 11 under *17 Conditions related to sexual health* are *HA61 Gender incongruence of childhood*, which naturally relates to prepubertal children, and *HA6Z Gender incongruence, unspecified*, which is a catch-all category. The DSM also includes a diagnosis of *Transvestic Disorder* to diagnose those people who have sexual arousal associated with cross-dressing and, crucially, significant distress associated with it. Similarly the historic ICD 10 included (*F60–F69*) *Disorders of adult personality and behaviour/F64 Gender identity disorders/F64.1 Dual-role transvestism*; (*F60–F69*) *Disorders of adult personality and behaviour/F65 Disorders of sexual preference/F65.1 Fetishistic transvestism*, for those people who cross-dressed and did not experience arousal or did experience arousal, respectively.

There is a strong argument against including diagnoses of transvestitism in current diagnostic manuals, not least the difficulty of determining what constitutes cross-dressing in contemporary fashions. There is, of course, an argument relating to distress – but why then list this possible cause of distress when we do not list other causes? We might imagine a Financial Insufficiency Disorder for example – whereby a patient is distressed due to having too little money. Transvestitism was retained in the DSM 5 because removing it was seen as being a "public relations disaster for psychiatry" (Spitzer, 2005 cited in Kleinplatz & Moser, 2005, p. 137). Nonetheless, some years later the World Health Organisation decided it could weather such disaster and has not included any 'transvestitism' diagnoses in the contemporary ICD 11.

Formulation

Diagnosis alone is, of course, insufficient in this field (and indeed in many fields to do with human beings living in the world) because a diagnosis pays little mind to the life of the person surrounding the criteria of the diagnosis. For example, a person might meet the criteria for *Gender Incongruence* detailed earlier but have an unaccepting family and be at risk of homelessness. Both of these things will impact upon the way that person is able to express their gender. Diagnoses can also be somewhat procrustean. Historically, this was notable for non-binary people who were not included under *F64.0 Transsexualism*. It is imperative, therefore, to consider the person in a holistic manner and only then to apply any diagnoses (if needed) as they fit to that formulation – rather than trying to fit the patient into the available diagnoses (cf. BPS, forthcoming 2021).

An Example of a Specialist Assessment

We will now consider an example specialist assessment. Naturally this will be adapted according to individual patient circumstances.

---

[9] We have used diversity in this book, rather than 'variant', as *diversity* is the more common term – we have ethnic diversity, not ethic variance. Variance also rather calls into question, variance from what? It rather presupposes a white, cisgender, heterosexual, able-bodied norm against which everything is measured and found to be 'varying'.

Introduction

• What does the client want from seeing you?

Some clients don't know, of course. When they do, it can be worth getting specifics, as clarity is vital so as not to make assumptions and then refer for the wrong thing. There is a surprising diversity of wishes, where sometimes both clinicians and clients assume there is only one 'pathway'.

• What is the client's gender identity?

Clients may have a label for this, or they may not. While, as noted earlier, gender is not a spectrum, it can be useful to consider it as one for the purposes of getting a rough feeling as to the gender of non-binary people. Are they more male, more female, both, neither – a fixed point, a range? (See Chapter 1, *Introduction*.)

Some people feel unable to say what their gender identity is because they are trying to accommodate the fact they feel unable to come out because of their fear of other people's reactions. Here the *Desert Island Question* can be helpful (it is worth asking for the client's forbearance before using this). This question is something like this:

> Imagine you have crashed down on a deserted desert island while flying on your own. You are fine, but you know, because of the instrument readings when you crashed, that you will not ever be found. You have enough provisions, desalination equipment, and the such to survive; and indeed you were transporting many different clothes, appliances, etc., such that you can live in whatever gender you choose – on your own – for the rest of your life. The question is: How do you live?

After having used this hypothetical example to obtain their internal gender identity, we can *then* bring the client back to what is stopping them from realising their gender in their real life.

• What are the client's preferred pronouns?

Aside from *Dr, Professor,* and so on (technically an honorific), if people identify as female these will usually be *she* and *Ms, Miss, Mrs*. And if male, *he* and *Mr*. For non-binary people *Mx* and singular *they* are most common.

• Has the client taken any steps to align their presentation with their gender?

This could include a change of name (it can be useful to find out why they chose it) and ID documents, any physical treatments such as hormones, surgeries, hair removal, clothing changes, and so on. Some people may be concerned about other people's reactions if they change their presentation; this can be addressed using the psychotherapeutic techniques detailed in Chapter 10, *Psychotherapy.*

• Has the client told anyone about their gender?

Coming out about one's gender, especially in the context of support, is associated with an improvement in mental and social functioning; indeed this improvement is in excess of that associated with hormones (Başar & Mutlu 2019) – of course both hormones and social transition can create an even larger effect.

Keeping one's gender secret can lead to distress, and difficulties later. For example, if a grandparent cannot be told about a client's gender, what will happen if they become ill, need to be visited by the patient, and the patient has a beard or breasts – will they then be told when they are unwell? There is never a 'right time', but generally engaging with the hard part of transition – telling others – creates good effects, and it often is far less of an issue than patients are 'certain' it will be. Indeed, aside from people one is intimate with, many people simply do not care very much when someone transitions. There are always some discriminatory idiots of course, but fortunately these seem to be relatively rare, even if abhorrent when it does occur. [10]

Gender History

- How old was the client when they first felt some degree of unhappiness with their gender?
- How old was the client when they first wore clothes not normally worn by that birth-assigned gender?
- When did they decide to change their body to align with their gender?
- When did they come out about their gender to others?
- Why come to services about their gender at this time?

It is not uncommon for a life event such as a decade birthday, death of a parent, separation, or the like to have acted as a trigger.

Sexual History

- Has the patient ever had a sexual encounter?

Do bear in mind that some people may be asexual, and some who have had sexual encounters may not have had them consensually.

- If so, how old were they on the first occasion?

    Naturally do not assume all people – patients or partners – will be heterosexual or cisgender.

- Obtain a history of significant partners, including marriages or civil partnerships and the conception of any children.

Of course again, be careful not to assume people are heterosexual or monogamous. People may be attracted to different genders, or irrespective of gender, and may be consensually non-monogamous.

- What is the client's current sexuality?

This can be complex and should be recorded. To get a simple additional idea, it can be worth asking how they would tick a box on a government form.

- Are they using a body part for sexual contact which they wish to change?

When this is the case, it is important to consider with the client both the costs and benefits of any change.

- Is there any fetishism?

People have a great many things they enjoy sexually. Provided they are consensual, there is little to trouble the psychiatrist or a psychologist. The key issue here is where there is erotic arousal associated with a change of gender role. In this case, see *Differential Diagnoses or Formulations for Gender Diversity* in this chapter.

Family History

- Has the client been adopted?

This is useful to avoid misinterpreting familial risk factors such as stroke, thromboembolic disease, depression, psychosis, and other conditions.

---

[10] Trans people have much higher rates of discrimination than cisgender people of course, just not to the level that would generally mean that transition into a more comfortable gender role would not be of net benefit.

- Draw a family genogram.

Do consider families of choice here.

- What is the mental and physical health of the client's family?
- Does the client have any [binary] trans or non-binary family members?

Trans family members can be a useful form of support and may have reassured the family that the sky won't fall in when someone transitions.

- What was the client's childhood and adolescence like?

We often ask this in the form of "In a sentence or phrase please describe your childhood" – otherwise you may need to settle down for: "Chapter the first. It was a rainy autumn day in late nineteen seventy-three when my parents . . . " Not unreasonable in some contexts, but not ideal when you have an hour to undertake a full assessment, and perhaps consequently determine treatment options.

- Was the client subject to physical or sexual abuse?

It can be worth asking this separately as some people will report a good childhood excluding abuse. Remember that sexual abuse does not preclude people from being trans because, tragically, a number of trans people are preyed upon because they are isolated precisely because they are trans.

Of course, we have a duty to report when people are at risk; naturally this must be done in the most sensitive and collaborative manner possible.

Physical History

- Does the client have any allergies?
- Does the client take any medications?

Self-medication, over-the-counter medication, and birth control should be specified as people often don't recount them in the list of medications taken.

- Does the client have any diagnoses?

We often phrase this as "do you have anything that you see your doctor for?" rather than diagnoses per se so that we pick up ongoing conditions which have associated check-ups. It is worth asking about developmental conditions such as ASC; psychiatric issues; as well as cardiac problems, strokes, clotting disorders, and migraines.

- Has the client had any operations?
- Does the client have any STIs?

We ask about these as they can affect some surgeries. The question may also act as a springboard for a discussion about safer sex. (See Chapter 8, *Sexuality, Relationships, and Reproduction*.)

- Does the client drink alcohol?

There are, of course, issues with liver function if a client is drinking to excess and the usual assistance should be offered. Additionally, if a client is masking their feelings through drinking to excess, it can be difficult to determine whether a transition is working for them.

- Does the client smoke?

Smoking raises thromboembolic risk and can be a contraindication to some hormones and surgeries. (See Chapter 3, *Physical Treatments for Trans People and Their Interactions with Psychiatric Treatments*.)

It is not uncommon for clients to lie about how much they smoke. It's helpful to explain the reasoning and to have assistance available with quitting. This is very hard and, of course, people do enjoy smoking. Many clients now vape, which is somewhat better than smoking tobacco; however, it can still be a contraindication to surgeries, especially if it contains nicotine, and again assistance with stopping vaping and taking nicotine in any form may be needed.

- Does the client take illicit substances?

As with use of alcohol, the use of illicit substances – especially if excessive – to manage mood is worrying and assistance should be given as usual. Again, when a person is masking gender dysphoria with illicit substances, it can be very hard to evaluate the progress of transition – certainly one would expect a reduction in illicit substance use as transition progresses.

- How tall is the client? How heavy are they?

A body mass index (BMI) over 30 can be a contraindication to some medical interventions. Do note that some patients hide their [gendered] body shape through being obese, and this group may have additional difficulties losing weight. It can be useful to encourage patients to see weight loss as part of a process of getting a body which is them – rather than one which is not.

Mental Health History

- Has the client had any contact with mental health services?

Not all clients will have had contact with a community mental health team, but some may have seen counsellors. Finding out about the precipitating factors to any mental health difficulties can be helpful in determining any assistance currently needed or situations which could be risky. If the client is still engaged with services, it can be useful to get names and contact details of any key contacts.

- Obtain any diagnoses or medications not mentioned before.
- Have there been any self-harm or suicide attempts?

It is important to get a history of self-harm and suicide attempts, including predisposing factors and triggers. Noting these and working with the client to manage them through the stresses and tribulations of transition can pay dividends. The usual assistance should be made available. Self-harm can be endemic in the context of gender diversity, as the dysphoria has such an embodied nature. Happily this often abates as transition progresses and more healthy coping strategies are found.

- Consider obtaining a mood score.

A general mood score from 0% "The worst you've ever felt" to 100% "The best you've ever felt" can be very helpful in evaluating progress. Of course, this scale is relative to the person rather than some absolute norm. Getting a zero may mean that action needs to be taken or may indicate that the person is trying to communicate distress and is not feeling listened to and so is resorting to hyperbole.

Forensic History

- Obtain the index offence and any other/older offences.

This is detailed in full in Chapter 6, *Forensic Settings*.

- Obtain the sentence and (if in prison) tariff and likelihood of parole.
- Obtain the names and contacts of staff in the secure estate, parole, police station, and so on.

- Assess risk.

The vast majority of trans people have never committed any offence. However, just as with any population – especially cisgender heterosexual males – some do perform criminal acts and should be managed accordingly.

Social Situation

- Confirm the client's address, where they reside, and if there is a chance of homelessness.
- Does the client have any savings or debt?

This is a good indicator of one element of practical support or stress available to them. There is no need to obtain the amounts.

- Does the client have any supportive friends? Do they know about the person's gender?

Many people do not particularly care about people's gender, especially after the initial period of coming out has passed. Sadly, however, some do, and some trans people can become isolated – perhaps especially if they are older, come from some black and minority ethnic communities, or have some other form of marginalisation. Some trans people form families of choice – a framily – and this should be respected.

People seldom wish to say they have no friends, so it can be useful to ask them if they have anyone who would lend them £20[11], or to whom they would lend £20. This gets around any awkward discussion as to whether the chap they buy their milk and bread from is really their friend (he may be), or is simply a grocer.

Educational and Occupational History

- Did the client go to school or college?
- Was the client bullied?

Bullying at school can significantly affect how people feel able to respond to their gender and any transition. If the client is still at school, the school should take robust action to stop bullying – being at school is not an excuse to allow abuse or assault which, outside of school, would be a disciplinary or police matter.

If the client has left school, they may need assistance to recognise that the (avoidance) behaviours which may have kept them safe in school need no longer apply and indeed may have now become a trap which is preventing them from flourishing.

- Did the client graduate?
- What did the client do next?
- Employment or occupational history.

This can be useful to see how settled or chaotic people's lives are and can lead to further avenues of exploration. It can also act as a trigger to see if the client has anything which they need help with such as filling out letters or attending appointments.

Formulation and Diagnosis

A formulation should be drafted which takes into account the detail obtained from the previous questions. Then a diagnosis may be made – if the person is trans or non-binary, not uncommonly it is *HA60 Gender Incongruence*.

---

[11] About the price of a reasonable pizza, coke, and dessert for our international readers.

Plan

A plan should be made, agreed and promulgated as necessary. It might include such things as the following:

- Further sessions of assessment? (with another clinician?)
- Refer elsewhere for other clinical assistance?
- Suggest community groups or resources?
- Refer for psychotherapy?
- Refer for speech and language therapy?
- Refer for hair removal?
- Refer for hormones?
- Refer for surgeries?
- Refer for other physical interventions?

Summary

The assessment of trans and non-binary people in a general setting is much the same as that for cisgender people, with mannered accommodation and a consideration of how the person's gender may inflect the presenting problem.

Specialist assessment of trans people is a more complex matter, usually best undertaken by a specialist in a gender identity clinic. The more complex the patient, the more experienced and senior the clinician should be. People with significant mental disorders and forensic histories should be seen by a consultant psychiatrist, consultant counselling psychologist, or consultant clinical psychologist.

In making assessments, we should ensure the very best rapport possible in our clinical setting. This will, almost invariably, include using the patient's preferred – correct – name and pronouns and ensuring that our broader services, including the elements outside of the clinical encounter, are inclusive and welcoming of gender diverse people.

Further Reading

British Psychological Society (BPS). (forthcoming 2021). *Guidelines for assessment, formulation, and diagnosis.* Leicester: British Psychological Society.

Richards, C., & Barker. M. (2013). *Sexuality and gender for mental health professionals: A practical guide.* London: Sage.

Richards, C., Bouman, W. P., & Barker, M. J. (eds.). (2018). *Genderqueer and non-binary genders.* London: Palgrave-Macmillan.

World Health Organization.(2019). HA60 Gender incongruence of adolescence or adulthood. In *International statistical classification of diseases and related health roblems 11.* Geneva: WHO.

References

American Psychiatric Association (APA). (2013a). *Diagnostic and statistical manual of mental disorders 5.* Washington, DC: American Psychiatric Association.

(2013b). *Gender dysphoria.* Washington, DC: American Psychiatric Association.

Başar, K., & Mutlu, E. (2019). *Improvement in mental well-being in individuals diagnosed with gender dysphoria with psychosocial support and hormone therapy: A prospective study.* Presentation to the European Professional Association of Transgender Health biennial conference. Rome, April.

British Psychological Society (BPS). (forthcoming 2021). *Guidelines for assessment, formulation, and diagnosis.* Leicester: British Psychological Society.

Herdt, G. (1996). *Third sex, third gender.* New York: Zone Books.

Kleinplatz, P. J., & Moser, C. (2005). Politics versus science: An addendum and response to Drs Spitzer and Fink. In D. Karasic & J. Drescher (eds.), *Sexual and gender diagnoses of the diagnostic and statistical manual* (DSM) (pp. 91–109). New York: The Haworth Press.

RCP sych (Royal College of Psychiatrists). (2013). *CR181 Good practice guidelines for the assessment and treatment of gender dysphoria.* London: Royal College of Psychiatrists.

World Health Organization. (1992). *International classification of diseases 10* (2nd ed). Geneva: WHO.

(2019a). *ICD11: Classifying disease to map the way we live and die.* Retrieved 16 May 2019 from www.who.int/health-topics/international-classification-of-diseases

(2019b). HA60 Gender incongruence of adolescence or adulthood. In *WHO international statistical classification of diseases and related health problems 11.* Geneva: WHO.

World Professional Association for Transgender Health (WPATH). (2011). *Standards of Care for the health of transsexual, transgender and gender nonconforming people* (7th ed). Minneapolis MN: WPATH.

World Professional Association for Transgender Health (WPATH). (forthcoming 2021). *Standards of Care for the health of transsexual, transgender and gender nonconforming people* (8th ed). Minneapolis MN: WPATH.

Physical Treatments for Trans People and Their Interactions with Psychiatric Treatments

Introduction

This chapter considers the extent to which trans folk need any adjustment to the pharmacological and physical therapies used in the treatment of coincidental mental illness or disorder as a result of existing endocrine treatment for gender dysphoria. Conversely it also considers the impact hormones and surgeries commonly used in the management of gender dysphoria may have on the treatments commonly used to treat mental illness.

The best approach is first to consider the endocrine treatment itself because if its aims, principles, and nature are properly understood the subsequent advice regarding psychotropic drugs is rendered logical and intelligible, and it becomes possible to extrapolate to other pharmacotherapeutic proposals that have not been covered or have yet to be developed.

The broad, overarching principle behind all endocrine treatment for trans folk is that of changing the patient's hormonal milieu so that it matches the gender identity of the patient. For the vast majority of patients this will mean a hormonal profile that matches the sex they were *not* assigned at birth; however, for a smaller number of patients with a non-binary gender identity (that is a gender other than male or female – see Chapter 1, *Introduction*), the desired hormonal profile will lie somewhere between these two points.

It should be noted that neither of these two points – a typically 'male' or 'female' hormonal profile – can reasonably be thought of as in any way extreme or unusual; they are simply the hormonal profiles of the rest of the [cisgender] patients who are more usually seen in the psychiatric clinic or on the ward. Pharmacological or physical treatments for mental illness that are generally considered safe to give to a [cisgender] man or a woman will, therefore, be just as safe if given to a trans man or a trans woman. It is only rarely that such physical treatments need special consideration or adjustment on account of the patient's trans status.

It should be noted that not all trans people will wish to have cross-sex hormones, although many do. Further many trans people also wish to have surgeries, although again this is by no means invariably so. Certainly trans people should not be reduced to their surgical or hormonal status as this forms only a part of their body and life. The detail of the available surgeries, and their impact upon psychiatric and psychological care, will be discussed later. For now, we will content ourselves with noting that it is important to continue any medication a patient is already taking. For example, if a person has had an oophorectomy or orchidectomy, they will need some form of sex steroids to ensure adequate energy and mood in the short term, and to maintain bone mineralisation and reduce risk of diabetes in the medium to long term.

Hormonal Treatment for Trans Men

Sex-steroid production by the endocrine system of cisgender men is probably more complicated than is generally recognised by the general public or even most general medical practitioners. The monthly cycle and commonly associated emotional changes that are seen in cisgender women do not feature, and it is thus an easy mistake to infer that cyclical changes are correspondingly absent in cisgender men.

Oestrogen levels in cisgender men are rarely measured; when they are, they tend to lie somewhere at a steady level between 70 and 120 pmol/L. Testosterone, on the other hand, exhibits a daily cycle, levels being highest in the morning and lowest in the evening. In addition to this diurnal variation, there is a superimposed annual cycle, the mean of these daily oscillations being higher in the spring and the autumn.[1] Diurnal variation in testosterone levels in cisgender men is a phenomenon more marked in youth; as cisgender men age, the amplitude of the cycle decreases and the mean levels fall.

Broader physical health is an important factor as well, because if cisgender men are unwell or otherwise psychologically or physically stressed, there can be – for the duration of the illness or stressful event – a period when the testosterone cycle is generally suppressed so that it resembles that of a much older person. It is partly for this reason that a young cisgender man with influenza isn't interested in sex, his enthusiasm reviving as the last snuffles recede.

In young cisgender men, the peak testosterone (measured at about 9 a.m.) is about 30 nmol/L, whilst the trough, just before he goes to bed, might be 15 nmol/L. An older man might experience a peak of 25 nmol/L and a trough of 10 nmol/L. This goes some way to explaining why the priapic young chap who snatches a kiss on his way to work (regretting that there's not time for more) has, by the time he goes to bed, when there is actually time available, so often transformed into a seemingly un-(a)rousable couch potato.

These perceptible changes in libido aside, there is, truth be told, but little variation in psychological or physiological function seen across the normal range of cisgender male testosterone. There *are* measurable differences, in fact, but they are so small as not to matter in any but rather special circumstances, one example being Olympic sprinting in which the host country tends to hold the race first thing in the morning in the hope that the fractionally faster times that result will lead to a record being broken at those particular games.

Endocrine treatment for trans men therefore aims to elicit testosterone levels and range somewhere in the range seen in a young cisgender man. It produces a variety of masculinising changes which are welcomed by the trans man or trans-masculine non-binary person (with the exception of going bald which – in common with many cisgender men – is usually unwelcome). Primary changes include soft tissue masculinisation such as redistribution of body fat away from the hips and chest[2] and towards the stomach, a coarsening of the skin, and the building of muscle mass. There will be male-typical body hair and, over time, the development of a full beard. The voice will 'break' into the male range. Their clitoris will grow significantly – generally enough for comfortable oral, but not anal or vaginal sex. As (for adults) the epiphyses have capped at puberty, there will be no additional height gain, although over time there may be moderate bone

---

[1] Tennyson was actually right when he said that in spring a young man's fancy lightly turns to thoughts of love (or at the very least a bit more sexual activity).

[2] Most trans men prefer their chest to be referred to as a chest, even if they have 'breasts' having not [yet] had a bilateral mastectomy and associated chest recontouring.

thickening due to the increased muscle mass. With prolonged use, their vagina may become dry (the usual lubricants can be used) and lose elasticity (an oestrogen pessary which largely only affects the tissue of the vagina can be prescribed to mitigate this). While many trans-masculine people do not wish to use their vagina, some do; as such, sexual health matters are naturally important (see Chapter 8, *Sexuality, Relationships, and Reproduction*). Interestingly, there is also fairly consistent anecdotal evidence that trans men feel the cold less than before starting testosterone.

There is often a sense of 'drive', sexuality and aggression increase, and the need to cry lessens. Mood often improves markedly, although this is usually not to do with a pharmacological mechanism, but rather because the person is able to present themselves as themselves in the world. This mood increase can result in stabilisation which mitigates some of the increased aggression; however, for patients with aggression as part of their risk profile, further monitoring and/or management is usually warranted. Psychiatrists and psychologists should be cautious of deferring treatment with testosterone solely on the basis of risk, as trans men frustrated by lack of treatment may well prove more of a risk than a contented trans man treated with testosterone. As always, careful consideration of the individual patient is paramount.

A variety of preparations of testosterone may be taken. Oral testosterone treatment is eschewed because it is associated with hepatocellular carcinoma, so most trans men are treated either with intramuscular testosterone injections or topical testosterone. Intramuscular testosterone injections given at the outset of treatment in a gender identity clinic tend to be in shorter-acting formats (examples are Sustanon, Virormone, or testos-terone enanthate) and need to be given so that the peak testosterone level, measured a week after the injection is given, is somewhere between 25 nmol/L and 30 nmol/L and the trough testosterone, measured immediately prior to the injection, is somewhere between 10 nmol/L and 15 nmol/L. The frequency required to achieve these figures varies a bit between patients but is usually three-weekly or four-weekly, and very rarely fortnightly.

Sometimes, when patients have been established on intramuscular testosterone for some time and often shortly before discharge from a gender identity clinic, shorter-acting intramuscular testosterone injections are replaced with longer-acting preparations. The best known of these is Nebido, which is usually given every twelve weeks. Only the trough testosterone is generally measured, immediately prior to the injection, and should be somewhere between 12 nmol/L and 20 nmol/L.

All the methods of administration and levels of testosterone detailed here usually stop the menstrual cycle (generally much to the patient's relief) but nonetheless cannot be relied upon as contraception and so conventional contraceptive measures should continue to be deployed if there is any risk of pregnancy. Progesterone-only hormonal methods, a progesterone-eluting IUD, or barrier contraception seems best. It bears repeating that STI risk remains the same and that barrier and other methods will be necessary. Trans men who wish to become pregnant must stop testosterone for a significant period beforehand – a process which is best undertaken under the care of an endocrinologist.

It should be noted that trans men treated with intramuscular testosterone have the same variation in testosterone levels over a three- or four-weekly period (or twelve-weekly period on Nebido) that cisgender men have on a daily basis. Consequently, no great emotional or psychological variation is expected or, generally speaking, evident. The only unwanted, hormonally mediated change in mental state that sometimes presents itself is a trans man reporting that he feels delicate, irritable, and tearful in the days before his injection is next due. This indicates that trough testosterone levels are inadequate and should prompt eliciting the advice of a gender identity clinic on adjusting the dose or dosing frequency.

Topical testosterone treatment is administered daily by the patient and aims to elicit a steady testosterone level somewhere in the normal daily range for a young cisgender man. Testosterone levels should be checked at least six hours after the medication has been applied, and the venepuncture site for the test should not be one to which the medication was earlier applied (failure to do either produces an artifactually high result). One of the cautions of using testosterone gels such as Testogel or Testim is that the patient must ensure that no gel touches women or children as, of course, the testosterone will be transferred – this can be understandably difficult in busy households or in inpatient settings. If the patient has poor self-care, it may be best to have a nurse-administered injectable preparation such as Sustanon or Nebido whereby the timing and dose can be controlled and there is no chance of accidental transfer.

Once established, monitoring either topical or injectable treatments in a general psychiatric setting is not difficult and consists of a twice a year measurement of testosterone level (peak and trough if short-acting intramuscular injections are being used; trough alone if long-acting injections; six hours after application if gel, as noted earlier) and full blood count including haematocrit, lipids, and liver function tests along with blood pressure and body mass index. Testosterone levels outside the desired range, deranged lipids or liver function tests, haematocrit in excess of 0.5, or hypertension all merit seeking advice from a gender identity clinic. A raised body mass index (BMI) responds to the conventional interventions for a raised BMI and does not require such advice.

The general physical risk profile for testosterone treatment is not significantly different from that of the general (untreated) population, and the precautions detailed here are to catch unusual cases, rather than expected difficulties in the usual course of things. That said, it is important to note that smoking and obesity both raise the cardiovascular risk profile for treatment with testosterone and therefore smokers should stop (vaping is acceptable for hormones, although not for genital surgeries) and people with very high BMIs should lose weight.

If the trans person retains their gynaecological organs while taking testosterone, there is, at the moment, thought to be a small risk of endometrial hyperplasia. Previously this risk was thought to merit hysterectomy in all cases, although this is no longer the case. Current advice is for a uterine ultrasound every two years. The test may be done abdominally if the person's anatomy allows. This can understandably be a distressing experience for a man, especially if there is an abuse history, so every courtesy and accommodation to his [male] gender should be afforded. If the patient is so overweight that abdominal ultrasonography isn't possible and a probe needs to be used, remember that the patient might prefer this to be placed rectally rather than vaginally. A uterus is a fairly large organ; as a result, it can be imaged in the general ultrasound department, the patient being accompanied to the appointment by a woman – nothing is more embarrassing than being a lone man in a gynaecological ultrasound department, drinking glass after glass of water, everyone knowing what that behaviour means.

Masculinising Hormonal Therapy for Non-binary People

Hormonal therapy for non-binary people does not differ markedly from that for binary trans people in that it involves initiating pubertal changes in the desired direction through the addition of exogenous hormones, and sometimes suppressing endogenous hormones. While binary trans people are usually happy with the full effects of puberty, non-binary people commonly wish for a limited range of types, or amount, of change. Of course pubertal changes occur in order and this cannot be changed hormonally; thus, a much deeper voice but no facial or body hair is not possible. The options are to use a 'full' dose and then stop when the desired changes have occurred or to use a reduced dose such that changes happen a little more slowly. However, in all cases patients need to recognise that it is not a 'menu' – one cannot pick and choose but rather must decide when in the process of puberty they would like to stop. In addition, the patient should be aware that after stopping, some changes such as body fat would revert, although characteristics like facial hair and vocal changes would remain. In addition, patients will need some form of sex steroid; accordingly, if they have been gonadectomised, they will need to decide if they would like a low maintenance dose of sex steroid of their sex assigned at birth or that of the other sex.

Hormonal Treatment for Trans Women

Feminising hormonal treatment for trans women also affects soft tissue predominantly. It will redistribute body fat from the abdomen and towards the breast and hips which will have a wider appearance, although the pelvis itself will not change. Mammary glands will develop, and the breasts will usually fall into the standard female range in terms of size, although they may appear smaller against the trans woman's (or trans-feminine person's) proportionally larger thorax. Her breasts may be induced to lactate and indeed some trans women have breastfed babies. Her skin will soften, and she may have erectile problems. Hair previously lost from the head will not regrow, and body and facial hair will need to be removed using laser or electrolysis – an expensive and often painful process. There are no vocal changes if the voice has 'broken' in puberty, but speech therapy and sometimes surgeries can be used to address this. She may feel more 'emotional', but mood improves and, interestingly, sexual drive often increases alongside a marked decrease of testosterone into the female range. This is because she is more at ease in her body and self and therefore naturally feels more sexual.

Of course, in cisgender women, testosterone levels do not vary significantly or cyclically and normally lie below 3 nmol/L but can be elevated to as high as 7 nmol/L if the woman has polycystic ovarian syndrome. Oestrogen levels, by contrast, vary in a complex monthly cycle with a trough of about 400 pmol/L and a peak which can, briefly, be as high as 1000 pmol/L. The physiological and emotional changes associated with this cycle should be known well enough to the reader as to not require describing again here.

Endocrine treatment for trans women therefore aims to elicit a steady oestradiol level somewhere between 400 pmol/L and 600 pmol/L, which is about the average level across the cycle in a cisgender woman. Because the risk of hepatotoxicity is very low, treatment is usually oral although occasionally, in patients who metabolise oestrogen particularly quickly, topical preparations are used because the number of tablets required to elicit the necessary levels becomes unwieldy and expensive, and it is simply cheaper and easier (but not safer, in the ordinary population) to utilise the topical route of delivery.

The dose of oral oestradiol required to elicit a serum oestradiol level between 400 pmol/L and 600 pmol/L varies quite a bit between individual women – with larger women, unsurprisingly, often requiring larger doses to achieve this. A typical dose might be 6 mg of oestradiol valerate each day; however, some trans women require up to 10 mg a day.

Pharmacists sometimes express alarm at the 'high doses' that are required, drawing a parallel with hormone replacement therapy for postmenopausal cisgender women. This is a false comparison, though, since the appropriate comparison is with younger cisgender women with premature ovarian failure, and the easy but false assumption made is that higher doses automatically lead to dangerous, higher levels. With any patient, or almost any medication for that matter, what matters is not the dose but rather the levels present in the patient's bloodstream. In most clinical settings, for almost any medication, the dose taken by the patient is being used as a convenient, proxy measure for blood level in the absence of the actual level itself. The degree of care and exactitude used in treating trans women with oestrogen is rather higher than this and consequently more, not less, reassurance should follow.

Other preparations include oestrogen gels such as Sandrena 0.5 mg to 1 mg sachets daily with bloods taken four to six hours after application (the gel should not be applied on the arms) or Estradot or Everel patches between 100 mcg and 200 mcg twice weekly with bloods taken after forty-eight hours and prior to the new patch (on the same day). Patches and gels are not the preferred route of administration for the reasons outlined earlier but are sometimes used when the patient is not having adequate responses to 10 mg of oestradiol orally. It has been postulated that this is due to a 'first pass effect'; accordingly, a means of administration other than orally is considered.

For most trans women eliciting a serum oestradiol between 400 pmol/L and 600 pmol/L does not suppress testosterone to levels seen in a cisgender woman. To do so requires a quite separate and physiologically independent pharmacological process given in parallel with oestrogen dosing. For this, complete testosterone suppression requires the additional administration of a gonadotrophin-releasing hormone analogue (GNRHa), typically given by intramuscular injection every twelve weeks. Many trans women seen in a general psychiatric setting will already be established on a twelve-weekly gonadotrophin-releasing hormone analogue injection and all that is required is for it to be continued. If it is to be started in such a setting, it should be after oestrogen levels are above 250 pmol/L. It should further be noted that for two weeks after the first injection (and only the *first* injection), a brief but marked rise in testosterone often precedes a precipitous fall. For this two-week period *only*, the trans woman will additionally need to be given cyproterone acetate at a dose of 50 mg a day to block the effects of this transient testosterone surge. Failure to prescribe the cyproterone acetate isn't dangerous but does condemn the trans woman to a fortnight of feeling, as one patient put it, "really horribly like a sweaty teenage boy with an endless erection and acne". This is not a pleasant proposition when one is a teenage boy – for a [trans] woman it may lead to risks associated with significantly lowered mood.

On some occasions, trans-feminine people require only partial suppression of testosterone. If this is the case, it is achieved with finasteride at a 5 mg daily, which is anecdotally (although, if you will, strongly anecdotally) associated with reduction in capital hair loss – an important intervention in this patient group who have fewer congenital cues of femininity. Such treatment can safely be continued in a general psychiatric setting provided liver function tests are normal.

It is important to note that in gender medicine the only role for cyproterone acetate is as testosterone receptor blockade in the two weeks after a gonadotrophin-releasing hormone analogue has first been given. It has no role other than this and should not be used in the longer term because such use is associated with depression, lethargy, fatigue, deranged liver function tests, and meningioma formation. Cyproterone acetate has never been licensed for use in human beings in the United States because it was believed to be too toxic. Patients seen in a general psychiatric setting who are found to have been self-medicating with cyproterone acetate should be advised to cease immediately, and the advice of a gender identity clinic as to the wisdom of ongoing prescribing of an appropriate medication should be sought.

While the use of oestrogens in trans women and trans-feminine people is generally very safe, thromboembolic risk is raised and accordingly smoking and obesity will need to be addressed. Additionally, those people with a history or familial risk of stroke or migraine should be assessed and possibly managed by an endocrinologist and may need to be moved to patches or gels. There is some suggestion that in older age, women should be moved from oral oestrogens to patches or gels or to have their hormones stopped altogether. This advice was largely based upon studies of cisgender women; it seems that for trans women, it is monitoring, rather than a change in preparation or cessation, which is reasonable in most cases.

There is some concern of a raised risk of cancers, including breast cancer, although it does not seem that this has proved to be the case in this population. Naturally the usual self-checking and medical screening procedures detailed later should be employed as appropriate.

Once established on a hormonal regimen, monitoring of BMI and blood pressure along with blood tests for oestrogen, testosterone, liver function tests (LFTs), and prolactin are usual – the latter to catch the extremely rare risk of a prolactinoma developing.

Feminising Hormonal Therapy for Non-binary People

Feminising hormonal therapy for non-binary people proceeds analogously to that for masculinising therapy detailed earlier, in that it is a matter of inducing puberty and stopping when the [possible] desired changes have occurred.

Screening for Trans People

Aside from the blood tests detailed elsewhere in this chapter, in most instances screening for trans people will occur in precisely the same way as for cisgender people, with only administrative adaptations needed – simple courtesy and respectful treatment with business as usual will be quite sufficient. Attention should be paid to the physical characteristics of the person as it is these which need screening and treating, rather than to gender – which should simply be respected for rapport. Naturally, people under psychiatric or psychological care should be facilitated to undertake such screening. The Cancer Research UK (2019) and the NHS (2019) have produced some excellent trans-specific guidelines for UK practice, and the following recommendations are summarised and adapted from them.

Population-based Screening

Trans people will be called according to the gender they register with their healthcare provider, and not necessarily their anatomy – accordingly due adaptations should be made.

Cervical Cancer

Anyone with a cervix should be screened every three years from age 25, as they are at risk of cervical cancer. The screening should also check for human papillomavirus (HPV). People AFAB registered as male will not be called and should be assisted both to attend and to make the process more comfortable and respectful of their gender. Patients should tell their doctor if they are taking testosterone and if they are still menstruating to ensure the test is accurate. Naturally people without a cervix need not be screened.

Breast Cancer

People with breasts should participate in breast screening from age 50 every three years until age 70. Only those registered as female with their primary care doctor will be called, and accommodation for those registered as male should be made. Patients who have had breast implants will need to tell the radiographer so the correct technique can be used.

People who have chest surgery to construct a masculine chest contour will still have some tissue remaining (the procedure is different from a radical mastectomy for cancer), but their risk is lower and mammography is usually not possible. Consequently other means of diagnosis should be undertaken if symptoms are present.

Bowel Screening

Population-based screening for bowel cancer does not differ by gender and is therefore the same for trans and non-binary people as it is for cisgender people. However, a person who has had a colo-vaginoplasty should let their physician know such that adaptations to practice and diagnosis can be made.

Abdominal Aortic Aneurysm

People registered as male with their primary care physician in the United Kingdom will be called for screening at age 65. Those people assigned male at birth – irrespective of transition or oestrogen treatment – are thought to be at risk, and so those registered as female who will not be called should be accommodated appropriately. There is some debate around whether people AFAB who are older than age 65 and who take testosterone – trans men and trans-masculine non-binary people – are at greater risk than cisgender women; accordingly, patients may well seek screening individually, or their physician may give serious consideration to making individual arrangements.

Specific Screening for Trans People

Some literature suggests that a few trans men and AFAB non-binary people who take testosterone develop a thickened endometrium which can increase the risk of endometrial cancer, although the literature is not clear at present. Previously the recommendation was to have a hysterectomy, but this is now not the case. Instead, the current recommendation is for people who have not had a hysterectomy for other reasons to have a pelvic ultrasound every two years.

While not used in the NHS aside from the first two weeks of GNRHa to offset the androgen flare, cyproterone acetate is sometimes offered to trans women and AMAB non-binary people in other settings to lower testosterone. It has a small increased risk of meningiomas.

Self-medication by Trans Folk

Many patients seen in psychiatric outpatient settings or admitted as an inpatient are taking medication purchased from the internet or obtained from any of a variety of other sources, not uncommonly because of the unconscionable wait to see a gender specialist caused by chronic under-resourcing of services. Whether such medication should simply continue to be prescribed at all is a question considered elsewhere (see WPATH 2011; forthcoming 2020); if it is, it should at least be rendered as safe as possible.

Self-medication with testosterone isn't so often seen and when it is tends to feature topical gels rather than intramuscular preparations. Trans men who self-medicate in this way often use excessive doses of testosterone, not knowing that very high serum testosterone levels activate metabolic pathways which are normally quiescent; those pathways convert the excess testosterone into oestrogen. The oestrogen so produced often causes griping, premenstrual-type pains, the response to which is a panicked further increase in the testosterone dose – effectively, it is like trying to put out fire with petrol. Patients self-medicating with testosterone need to have their serum testosterone levels measured and the dose adjusted accordingly.

Self-medication with oestrogen is commonly seen, the most frequent error being too high an oestrogen level established so rapidly that it has caused early ductal fusion in the breasts, resulting in the development of small, hard, conical-shaped breasts that will not grow any larger whatever the subsequent hormonal treatment. Patients self-medicating with oestrogen need levels measured and doses adjusted accordingly.

Self-medication with a gonadotrophin-releasing hormone analogue isn't commonly seen because these agents are expensive and require injecting. Instead, many patients present self-medicating with oral agents in an attempt to suppress testosterone. The most frequently encountered is probably spironolactone, which has some testosterone receptor antagonist properties. Spironolactone serves also to derange electrolytes, is associated with depression and diminished final breast size, and triples the risk of upper gastrointestinal haemorrhage. It is best discontinued for these reasons. Patients sometimes self-medicate with cyproterone acetate. As stated earlier, there are considerable side effects of this drug and it too is best discontinued.

Patients often self-medicate with progesterone or may suggest that this would be a useful medication to add. This is not the case. The endocrinology of human puberty doesn't feature progesterone until breast development has been completed, progesterone serving as it does to drive ductal readiness for breastfeeding rather than breast growth itself. Separately, massive long-term studies of hormone replacement therapy in cisgender women have shown that mixed oestrogen and progesterone therapy raises the risk of breast cancer whilst oestrogen-only therapy does not (as used by women who have had a hysterectomy and accordingly don't need progesterone to protect against uterine cancer). The advice for a cisgender woman with no uterus would be to take oestrogen only and the same advice applies to a trans woman for exactly the same reasons.

Interactions with Psychotropic Medication

The preceding preparatory preamble through the principles behind endocrine treatment for trans folk should make it clear that interactions should be refreshingly few, which is indeed the case. Any psychotropic medication which is known to work equally well in males and females (premenopausal and postmenopausal) can just as easily be given to a trans person in exactly the same way.

Psychotropic agents with dopamine antagonistic properties (largely antipsychotics) sometimes elevate prolactin in cisgender women and will do exactly the same in trans women and trans men. There may be lactation as a result, and it might be much more distressing to a trans man who still has breasts than to a cisgender woman. The slightly raised risk of a prolactinoma in trans women on oestrogens should be taken into account; however, cessation of oestrogen should not be the immediate consideration as this is associated with very significant decompensation.

Some psychotropic agents, including older anti-epileptic medication, act to induce cytochrome P450 and other drug metabolic pathways. As a result, higher than expected doses of oestrogen may be needed to elicit the desired oestrogen levels in trans women, just as cisgender women taking the same psychotropic medication sometimes need to take a double dose of the contraceptive pill to obtain a reliable contraceptive action.

Interactions with Non-prescribed Psychotropic Agents

Rather more needs to be said in connection with non-prescribed psychotropic agents, for it is here that risks abound. By far the most life threatening is tobacco, if it is smoked (as it almost always is, snuff having fallen out of favour a while ago now). Smoking greatly raises the risk of thromboembolic disease and, as stated above, thromboembolic risk rises also with oestrogen treatment. The combination of the two is a risk easily avoided by stopping either the oestrogen or the smoking – most patients would rather cease the second. Smoking also greatly raises the risk of polycythaemia (which carries many health risks) and testosterone raises red cell count also. The combination of the two is, again, a risk easily avoided and, again, most trans men would rather stop smoking than stop testosterone[3].

It should be noted that the common risk here is that of smoking, not of nicotine. Electronic cigarettes, nicotine chewing gum or patches, or indeed any other sort of nicotine substitution is much more compatible with hormone treatment (but not genital surgeries).[4] Using these products is also less expensive and more socially acceptable.

Cannabis, if smoked, carries all the risks of smoking and is thus incompatible with hormone therapy. If taken by another route, it is worthwhile noting that cannabis contains oestrogen receptor agonists; trans men smoking cannabis because they are 'stressed' by having breasts should be aware that they are, in fact, contributing to the very problems that are stressing them and ought to be made aware of the self-defeating nature of their coping strategy. Further, those who have a genetic loading for psychosis, because they are trans, are also under stress. If cannabis is added to this increased risk profile – especially potent strains now more common in some areas – there is a risk of the development of a psychotic illness.

This patient group similarly sometimes uses alcohol to manage stress. It is a potent liver enzyme inducer and hepatotoxin. Anything but modest alcohol use makes treatment with oestrogen or testosterone difficult to undertake as levels may vary wildly and raises the risk of hepatotoxicity.

---

[3] Sadly some patients misunderstand the nature of risk and say something to the effect that "My friend smokes/takes X/does Y, and he's OK, so I can take/do them too." An example of playing 'Russian roulette' can be a useful clarification here – explaining that simply because their friend happened to be OK when they pulled the trigger does not mean there is no risk to them doing so too.

[4] This is true at the time of writing, although there are the first rumblings of discontent on vaping and e-cigarettes from the medical community. The reader should, as always, check for the latest advice.

Fertility

Giving testosterone to people assigned female at birth or oestrogen to people assigned male at birth will affect fertility. Fertility loss is not guaranteed, and barrier methods of contraception should be employed where risk of unwanted pregnancy is possible.[5] Nonetheless there is also a significant risk of loss of fertility and a certain loss when orchiectomy or oophorectomy is undertaken. Accordingly, gamete storage should be considered (see Chapter 8, *Sexuality, Relationships, and Reproduction*).

Electro-Convulsive Therapy – ECT

Those taking gonadotrophin-releasing hormone analogue (GNRHa) while undergoing ECT will need an ECG due to the link to prolonged QT in some cases. In addition, the procoagulant anaesthesia can alter hormone metabolism and accordingly hormone levels and associated risks outlined earlier should be monitored and managed. Again, simply stopping hormones will almost certainly cause significant decompensation and should only be considered when absolutely necessary.

Trans-masculine Surgeries

Masculinising surgery includes a bilateral mastectomy and associated chest recontouring, which is by far the most common surgery requested by both trans men and trans-masculine non-binary folk. It allows the person to forgo the tight binder which has flattened their chest heretofore and so wear a light shirt in summer, go swimming, be intimate, and indeed often simply see themselves in the mirror comfortably.

Some chaps also request a hysterectomy and oophorectomy and phalloplasty or metoidioplasty (the creation of a phallus) along with a scrotoplasty. The metoidioplasty involves the clitoris getting larger under the effects of testosterone, the ligament holding it in place being released, and labial skin being used to wrap it to give bulk. It has the possibility of creating a urethra such that the chap can stand to urinate, although this naturally carries with it the risk of urinary incontinence if there are complications which cannot be resolved. A scrotum may be created (scrotoplasty) using labial skin, which uses the usual testicular implants which are available for men who have undergone orchiectomy. The resulting phallus is sensate, as the nerves and blood supply are retained, and will become erect with arousal and may be used for orally penetrative, but not usually vaginally or anally penetrative sex.

Some chaps instead opt for a phalloplasty, usually using a graft from the forearm, abdomen, or thigh depending on whether sufficient tissue is available, whether the chap can tolerate a forearm scar, the nature of sensation requested, and other surgical considerations peculiar to the individual. The phalloplasty creates a larger phallus, which some chaps prefer as it fills their underpants to give a larger contour. If the urethra is connected and routed through the phallus, the chap can stand to urinate, although again there may be complications leading to urinary incontinence. As it is a micro-surgical procedure to connect the nerves and blood vessels, the risk of loss of sensation and necrosis is greater, and sadly complications are not uncommon. Here again chaps may opt to have a scrotoplasty as detailed earlier, with the

---

[5] And we must be careful not to assume that unwanted pregnancy is not possible or is unlikely due to the person's trans status – a trans man or trans-masculine person who has sex with a cisgender man, for example (which is not uncommon), would certainly be at such risk.

clitoris usually buried at the base of the shaft of the phallus and still providing sexual sensation. A prothesis may also be included which has a reservoir in the abdomen, a pump in place of one testicle and an inflatable rod in the shaft of the phallus. Pumping one testicle allows the phallus to become hard for oral, vaginal, or anal sex; the rod can then be deflated by means of a button. Again, complications are possible, and not uncommon. Non-binary surgeries tend to be variations on these and are detailed by Ralph, Christopher, and Garaffa, as well as Bellringer, in Richards, Bouman and Barker (2018).

Complications for all surgeries include urinary incontinence, infection, and necrosis of the phallus. These are very much increased if the patient is obese or a smoker and so smoking cessation is required beforehand (with carbon monoxide–bound haemoglobin checks to ensure veracity) and a BMI of less than 31. Further, nicotine has been shown to poorly affect surgical outcomes and so the patient may also need to abstain from vaping [nicotine] prior to surgery. There are no particular contraindications to psychiatric treatments which cannot be managed by the surgical team if the patient is in a stable enough mental state.

Trans-feminine Surgeries

Trans-feminine surgeries may include augmentation mammoplasty, although this is very rare if feminising hormones are managed properly. Trans-feminine people may also wish to have facial feminisation surgery, which is (in our view erroneously) not available via the United Kingdom's NHS. This is often requested early on; however, after feminisation with oestrogens, many trans people elect not to pursue it after all, and some have a more modest request, rather than feeling the need to change 'whole cloth' to be 'legitimate'. Some people also request a reduction of their laryngeal prominence and/or vocal pitch surgery, although the pitch often reverts after some time and so the surgery is less common now than it once was. Some, but by no means all, request genital surgery.

Genital surgeries include orchiectomy either alone or with the creation of a vulva, clitoris, and feminine urethral opening. An orchiectomy naturally removes the need for exogenous androgen suppression, as adrenal androgens are, of course, insufficient in people assigned male at birth to reach the cisgender male range. Some, but not all, people who opt to have an orchiectomy with the creation of a vulva from scrotal tissue, clitoris from the glans, and feminine urethral opening, also opt to have a vagina to have vaginally penetrative sex.[6] The vagina is usually formed from the skin of the penis which is inverted. Additional skin from the scrotum may be used if there is insufficient penile skin due to circumcision, genetics, or GNRHa use early in puberty resulting in a small penis. Another option is to use tissue from the colon; however, as well as reported smell and continuous lubrication, this appears to fail after about 15 years necessitating repeat surgeries in younger patients. As with trans-masculine surgeries, for more information on the surgeries requested by non-binary folk, see Bellringer in Richards, Bouman and Barker (2018).

However created, the neo-vagina will need dilating with an acrylic dilator several times a day after surgery, lowering to just a couple of times a week once full recovery has occurred. This is vital throughout the person's life to keep the neo-vagina open so as to prevent stenosis and subsequent infection (see Chapter 8, *Sexuality, Relationships, and*

---

[6] As a side note, it is important on the rare occasions when one does discuss genitals not to refer to a vulva as a vagina. Difficulties can arise in instances such as these, as well as when discussing STI transmission, sexuality, and the like.

Reproduction). Complications again include urinary incontinence, infection, and necrosis of the neo-vagina as well as the risk of prolapse, which are very much increased if the patient is obese or a smoker and so smoking cessation is required beforehand (with carbon monoxide–bound haemoglobin checks to ensure veracity) and a BMI of less than 31. There are no particular contraindications to psychiatric treatments which cannot be managed by the surgical team if the patient is in a stable enough mental state.

General Surgical Considerations

It should go without saying that it is important not to reduce people to their genital status and not to ask about genitals or surgery unless it is absolutely necessary. That aside, considerations relating to surgery of those with mental health issues broadly relate to whether the patient is mentally robust enough to undergo surgery and can manage sufficient self-care to recover afterwards. With all people and all surgeries, post-surgical depression can occur, and this will need careful consideration and support in those with a depressive illness or risk of decompensation. This can be exacerbated in those cases where surgery was not successful, or in those unfamiliar with the look of a recent surgical site who may be distressed without realising that the appearance will change radically over the next several months. Medical reassurance that much will change and that even in cases where things have gone wrong, much can still be done irrespective of how it looks now can pay dividends.

Additionally, surgery can act as a psychological threshold for friends and family. In some cases, this is a positive thing as they believe it confers legitimacy on the trans person; however, in some cases they very unfortunately choose the surgical recovery period to disown the trans person with tragic results. In this instance, trans people should naturally be supported through both the surgery and the relationship problems. This is especially important because surgical outcomes can affect patient's consideration of their whole transition – with a catastrophising stance being a risk at this stage. Careful support, reassurance, and management may be necessary in this instance.

Regret

It is very rare for people to regret surgery. It is vastly less common than in the popular imagination, and regret rates are in line with many other types of surgery unrelated to gender. Regret of gender-related surgeries is almost invariably due to the person not being properly screened for surgery (see Chapter 2, *Assessment*) and having it undertaken in the private sector in countries with more lax criteria than the NHS in the United Kingdom. All people regretting surgery should be referred to the care of a gender identity clinic.

As stated earlier, regret is vanishingly rare; however, it is important to arrange things such that the patient, even if not regretting *that* they had surgery, does not have cause to regret *how* they had it. In some cases, surgery may need to be deferred until the patient is more psychologically stable, but this should be balanced against the stress of not receiving a needed surgery in a timely manner, and the very significant benefit receiving such surgery confers in terms of mental health (Bränström & Pachankis, 2019; Gijs & Brewaeys, 2007)

Other risks associated with surgery include the low energy and mood which occur when hormones are paused prior to surgery to reduce thromboembolic risk. This will abate after surgery when the hormones restart but can be stressful, especially as, of course, it occurs during the often anxious wait for the surgery itself.

Summary

There are no particular ongoing health issues for trans people beyond those of cisgender people throughout their life, provided they have appropriate screening, continue the hormonal regimen recommended by their endocrinologist, and dilate if necessary. Accordingly, if these matters are attended to, there are no especial ongoing issues for trans people with psychiatric conditions aside from the maintenance of the interventions already started. The only other consideration is that patients will not be registered under their birth-assigned sex but will still need screening appropriate to their anatomy; trans people with psychiatric illnesses which affect self-care may need assistance to access such services.

Beyond these relatively minor extra matters, we hope this chapter has reassured our colleagues that there is no need to be unduly wary of continuing or initiating gender-related treatments when people are being treated for a mental illness. Indeed, gender-related treatments often allow for better rapport and reduce stress, allowing for more effective treatment of mental illness.

Further Reading

Ettner, R., Monstrey, S., & Eyler, A. E. (eds.). (2016). *Principles of transgender medicine and surgery* (2nd ed.). New York: The Haworth Press.

Richards, C., Bouman, W. P., & Barker, M. J. (eds.). (2018). *Genderqueer and non-binary genders.* London: Palgrave-Macmillan.

References

Bränström, R., & Pachankis, J. E. (2019). Reduction in mental health treatment utilization among transgender individuals after gender-affirming surgeries: A total population study. *American Journal of Psychiatry*, 1–8. doi:10.1176/appi.ajp.2019.19010080

Cancer Research UK (2019). I'm trans or non-binary. Does this affect my cancer screening? Available from www.cancerresearchuk.org/im-trans-or-non-binary-does-this-affect-my-cancer-screening

Gijs, L., & Brewaeys, A. (2007). Surgical treatment of gender dysphoria in adults and adolescents: Recent developments, effectiveness, and challenges. *Annual Review of Sex Research*, *18*, 178–224.

NHS (2019). *Information for trans and non-binary people: NHS screening programmes.* https://assets.publishing.service.gov.uk/government/uploads/system/uploads/attachment_data/file/834656/Screening_for_trans_and_non-binary_people_Sept_2019.pdf

Richards, C., Bouman, W, P., & Barker, M. J. (eds.). (2018). *Genderqueer and non-binary genders.* London: Palgrave-Macmillan.

World Professional Association for Transgender Health (WPATH) (2011). *Standards of care for transgender and gender non-conforming people Version 7.* Minneapolis, MN: WPATH.

World Professional Association for Transgender Health (WPATH) (forthcoming 2020). *Standards of care for transgender and gender non-conforming people Version 8.* Minneapolis, MN: WPATH.

Mental Health Conditions

Introduction

In the World Health Organization's historic *International classification of diseases version 10* (WHO, ICD 10, 1992), and all earlier versions which considered the matter, gender dysphoria was termed 'Transsexualism' and classified in the section devoted to disorders of adult personality and behaviour. By the early twenty-first century, this placement came to seem increasingly inappropriate, not least because, notwithstanding prejudice towards trans people leading to depression and anxiety (Robles et al., 2016), the rates of psychopathology are no higher among trans people than among cisgender people (Colizzi, Costa, & Todarello, 2014; Hill et al., 2005; Hoshiai et al., 2010; Simon et al., 2011). Consequently the WHO has stated that the renamed Gender Incongruence is *not* a mental disorder (WHO, 2019a) and, in the *International statistical classification of diseases version 11* (WHO, 2019b) has been moved out of sections related to mental disorders and into the section devoted to *Conditions related to sexual health.*[1] The retention of any diagnosis at all differs from the debates surrounding the removal of homosexuality from the American Psychiatric Association's *Diagnostic and statistical manual* (DSM) in 1973 and from the ICD in 1992, in that same-gender attraction does not require any specific intervention and associated diagnosis, whereas under current arrangements, trans people seeking hormones or surgeries do.

Notwithstanding this pragmatic need for a [non-psychiatric] diagnosis, trans folk do not have a mental illness or disorder simply by virtue of being trans – and accordingly ought not to be treated as if they do. On the other hand, being trans does not magically confer some sort of immunity from all known forms of mental illness or disorder, and it is consequently perfectly possible for someone to be both trans and also, incidentally, to have exactly such an illness or disorder.

Trans folk share with the gay, lesbian, and bisexual population a slightly greater rate of some diagnosable mental disorders. The representation of increase is not even across the broad spectrum of diagnoses but rather a few, specific diagnoses that appear to be considerably over-represented whilst others are found only at population levels. Major

---

[1] There is much confusion relating to where gender diversity should be placed, if anywhere, both regarding the ICD and in terms of the NHS and healthcare in general. It could be considered to be developmental, psychological, endocrinological, surgical, or any number of other specialties, conditions, or diagnostic categories (or combinations thereof). This is, of course, a failure of our taxonomy, not a comment on the condition itself. The whole matter is reminiscent of the debates about the platypus in the early nineteenth century where nature was unduly forced into the extant cladistic understandings, until it was reluctantly accepted that our understanding had to adapt to the beautiful diversity of nature, rather than the other way around.

psychotic illness and major bipolar mood disorder do not seem to occur more commonly in the context of trans status than in the general population. Substance abuse disorders are, perhaps, a little more common, depressive disorders rather more frequently diagnosed, emotionally unstable personality disorder more frequently diagnosed in trans men, and the autistic spectrum conditions vastly more frequently diagnosed in all trans folk.

It is less than entirely clear what lies behind this particular and uneven pattern of diagnoses. At its simplest level, the increased rate of substance abuse and depressive disorders may well reflect minority or marginalisation stress as is the case in gay, lesbian, and bisexual folk. Further, if one follows the diathesis-stress model of mental illness, a person with a genetic loading towards mental illness who is placed under stress is significantly more likely to display symptoms, which can have a progressive outcome as they adversely affect the person's life in a vicious spiral. Naturally the stress of being trans in a too-often unaccepting world is precisely the form of stress which can precipitate such decompensation. This is not to say that people with mental illness should suppress their trans identity, as this will cause more, not less, stress and accordingly more decompensation (see Chapter 5, *Supporting Trans and Non-binary People in Mental Health Services*).

Another particular factor which may, in part, account for the increased rate of diagnosed depression and anxiety in trans folk is that they are rather more likely to be seeking medical intervention in the form of hormone treatment or surgery, and, as a general principle, the greater the amount of time one spends in the company of medical practitioners and clinicians – particularly psychiatrists or psychologists – the more likely one is to attract a diagnosis of depression. People who rarely visit a doctor seldom attract such a diagnosis, whatever their state of mind.

The vastly increased rate of a coincidental diagnosis of an autistic spectrum disorder is an exceedingly robust finding which has often been duplicated (Øien, Cicchetti, & Nordahl-Hansen, 2018). Indeed, so important is this coincidental diagnosis that an entire separate chapter of this book has been devoted to the intersection between gender dysphoria and autistic spectrum conditions (see Chapter 7, *Autistic Spectrum Conditions and Intellectual Disability*) and for that reason it will not be further considered here. Additionally, it is not the role of this book to explore the various competing hypotheses that attempt to explain this association, none of which is entirely convincing. Instead, this chapter concentrates on the diagnostic and therapeutic problems presented by the coincidence of mental illnesses and disorders with gender diversity.

Psychosis

It is entirely possible for a trans person to have or to develop a psychotic illness. The pharmacological treatment of such an illness is generally possible in exactly the same way as would apply if the person were not trans (see Chapter 3, *Physical Treatments for Trans People and Their Interactions with Psychiatric Treatments*). Rather, the difficulty lies in establishing a firm diagnosis relating to gender dysphoria in the context of psychosis and, should such a diagnosis be made, attempting to do useful therapeutic work with a trans person who is additionally psychotic.

It is not at all common for psychosis to present with a delusion regarding gender identity. Delusions and sometimes somatic hallucinations related to bodily alteration are a fairly common presentation of psychosis – often in the form of passivity phenomena – but the bodily changes which the patient reports are usually presented as a negative, unwanted occurrence imposed from outside the self or, more rarely, in a bland and neutral way. This can be distinguished from a desire for bodily change which has not yet occurred but is strongly wanted and which takes its origin in a sense of self, rather than anything imposed from outside the self.

It can sometimes be difficult to very clearly identify gender dysphoria in an individual who is floridly psychotic; however, for anyone in such a state, the major health need is the active treatment of the psychosis. If gender dysphoria and psychosis are independently present, then as the psychosis wanes the gender dysphoria remains unaltered and becomes consequently more prominent, often taking a less disordered, more typical, form of presentation.

Trying to address gender dysphoria in a patient who has an additional psychotic illness is an enterprise in which it is best to get on the right footing from the outset. Patients with a long-standing illness very often fear that their psychiatric illness means that their gender dysphoria will not be taken seriously and, sad to say, all too often their fears in this regard are justified. Instead, we recommend gaining a consultation with a gender identity clinic consultant psychiatrist or consultant psychologist as soon as is practicably possible to determine any diagnosis and collaborate on any treatment recommendations (see Chapter 5, *Supporting Trans and Non-binary People in Mental Health Services*).

It is very often helpful to make clear that when addressing gender dysphoria in the context of *any* chronic illness – be that illness physical or mental – the best progress can only be made if the patient does their utmost to cooperate with the clinicians treating the additional chronic illness. Accordingly, if the patient has type one diabetes or asthma, it will not be possible to properly address the gender dysphoria if they are repeatedly admitted to hospital with diabetic crises or acute respiratory distress because they have neglected to take their insulin or refused to use their inhaler respectively. In an exactly analogous way, it will not be possible to address properly the patient's gender dysphoria if they are repeatedly admitted to hospital with psychiatric crises or are too thought disordered to manage in day-to-day life as a result of neglecting to take the treatment for the additional psychiatric illness. The key point is that no distinction is made because the patient's additional illness is psychiatric – the same conditions would apply for a chronic physical complaint.

If the psychotic illness is under good control, assistance with gender dysphoria in the form of physical treatments is generally possible, although frequent hurdles are difficulties with smoking cessation and weight loss and the tendency of negative symptoms to impair reliable compliance with hormone treatment – particularly intermittent injections of a gonadotrophin-releasing hormone analogue. In many regards, a well-circumscribed delusional disorder tends to be the psychotic illness that offers least impediment to successfully managing gender dysphoria.

We should note here that if people are transgender prior to requiring treatment for psychosis – whether this is an initial presentation of psychosis or a new episode, under no circumstances should the person be de-transitioned while addressing their psychosis. This will almost inevitably lead to disengagement from treatment and marked decompensation (see Chapter 5, *Supporting Trans and Non-binary People in Mental Health Services*).

Major Mood Disorder

People with a pathologically elevated mood can present with what can superficially seem to be gender dysphoria, but the presentation tends to be flamboyant and sexualised. A return to a euthymic state is usually accompanied by a corresponding diminution in this behaviour and any declared gender dysphoria. In those trans folk with an additional bipolar disorder, mania is generally not accompanied by any change in gender identity, although personal presentation becomes much as one would expect from elevated mood, with the equally expected decline to a more socially conventional presentation, in exactly the same gender role, as mood returns to normal. As with psychotic disorders, a major issue is that of gaining the confidence of the patient that the gender dysphoria will be taken seriously. A frequent additional hurdle is the patient being too psychomotor retarded to comply properly with endocrine treatment at times of depressed mood or too chaotic at times of elevated mood – at exactly the time when there are frequently very forceful demands for premature increases in treatment, surgical interventions, and so forth.

Substance Abuse

The rate of substance abuse in the context of gender dysphoria is, perhaps, a little higher in the population of patients seeking treatment at a gender identity clinic. To a considerable extent, substance abuse in such patients represents self-medication of the psychological distress caused by gender dysphoria; it is refreshing to note that addressing the gender dysphoria is often accompanied by a gratifying remission in the preceding substance abuse. However, it can be difficult to assess people for gender dysphoria if they have significant substance misuse as their general functioning, and the substances they are taking, can mask response to treatment. Therefore reduction and abstinence may need to be sought as part of assessment.

This being said, chronic substance abuse continues in some patients despite their gender dysphoria being addressed; for such patients, exactly the same advice applies. It will be necessary for them to have their opiate addiction (or whatever the substance abused) under good control if treatment is to progress.

In those patients with a history of a chemical dependence syndrome which has remitted when their gender dysphoria has been addressed, it is important for the patient to know that the phenomenon of reinstatement applies just as much to them as it does to anyone else who has had a dependence syndrome. Returning to substance use, including recreationally, is liable to lead to speedy relapse and the reinstatement of substance misuse. Surgical interventions related to gender dysphoria are particularly important since very often opiate analgesia is part of the process and risks triggering reinstatement as a result. Patients with a history of opiate dependence syndrome are well advised to make the surgeon and anaesthetist aware of this in advance. It can be helpful if they agree in advance that their analgesia is best titrated according to the judgement of their clinician with regard to necessity, rather than their statement of need at the time. It is wise for them to be discharged home with medication that does *not* contain opiates; high-dose non-steroidal anti-inflammatory agents in combination with paracetamol can be a surprisingly effective and often neglected substitute in these circumstances.

Social Phobia and Other Anxiety Disorders

A diagnosis of social phobia is more common in the context of a gender identity clinic and may often reflect one feature of an undiagnosed autistic spectrum condition. If it is found in isolation (an autistic spectrum condition having been excluded), it can be particularly difficult for the trans person affected because of the inhibiting effect it has on achieving a change of social gender role. Usefully, social phobia in this context responds in exactly the same way as does social phobia in any other; as a result, local psychiatric services which are able to address social phobia in the general population should also be able to address social phobia in the context of gender dysphoria – see Chapter 10, *Psychotherapy*, for more detail on how this may be addressed. Accordingly, there is no requirement for specialist services at a gender identity clinic to address this aspect, even though local services might initially maintain that this is the case. We should note that for those with social phobia, and indeed many trans people in general who are more at risk of staying indoors, there are very high rates of vitamin D deficiency, and testing and treatment for this may prove necessary.

Depression

Trans people are more likely to be depressed than cisgender people. This is in part because being trans is a bit harder than being cisgender – for example, there is often a need for hormones, surgeries, and so forth; well-fitting clothes can be hard to find; the vision in the mirror doesn't match one's self-image, and so on. Prejudice and discrimination can understandably cause low mood – including with family and relationships (see Chapter 8, *Sexuality, Relationships, and Reproduction*), as well as the general public (see Chapter 9, *Legal and Religious Aspects*). It is important to stress, however, that this is not invariably so. When trans people are psychologically robust and/or well supported – and especially if they are not subjected to minority/marginalisation stress – they can live entirely content lives.

The clinical job regarding low mood in trans people, therefore, is commonly either to act as a bridge to a better state of affairs – until the person is able to come out, for example or to mitigate the distress of a prejudiced world to some extent. In both instances, pharmacological and/or therapeutic interventions may be considered. This should not generally need to be a specialist matter as common antidepressants can safely be used with the usual hormones and anti-androgens (see Chapter 3, *Physical Treatments for Trans People and Their Interactions with Psychiatric Treatments*); psychotherapeutic techniques which work on depression for other matters can usefully be used here too (see Chapter 10, *Psychotherapy*).

Lastly, we should note that there can be a tendency, on the part of both patients and doctors, to assume that gender-related physical interventions will act as something of a panacea – and indeed they can but *for gender*. The patient who is living in poverty with a chronic health condition will still be doing so after a change of role and associated treatments – they may be able to manage those things a little better, but their lot will likely still lead to depression. Surprisingly, this can come as a disappointment to both the patient and those around them. This is, of course, not to say that the treatments have 'failed' but rather that they have only acted in the domain in which they can – that of gender. Further, upon transition one often swaps one set of problems for another – for example, in a sexist society one may now feel able to wear a skirt to work but may also get listened to less at meetings.[2]

Emotionally Unstable Personality Disorder/ Personality Disorder – Borderline Pattern

This disorder – or a condition of complex PTSD if one is so minded – is a more frequent diagnosis at first presentation to a gender identity clinic in trans men than it is in trans

---

[2] This really is something which is commonly reported by trans patients. There is an illustrative, if possibly apocryphal, story of two doctors overheard discussing an eminent trans doctor at a conference – one said, "She's very good, isn't she?" The other replied, "She is, but you should have heard her brother."

women. One decidedly plausible explanation for this phenomenon is that if an individual gets into physical fights, drinks alcohol to excess, engages in random acts of minor vandalism, and displays a fair amount of sexual promiscuity, then they are liable, if female, to attract a diagnosis of an emotionally unstable personality disorder, whereas if they were male, they would instead be viewed as a typical, if annoying, teenage boy. The over-representation of this diagnosis in trans men may therefore represent nothing more than them behaving in a typically masculine manner in a setting where others perceive them as female.

There is also the sad fact that trans people are more subject to verbal, physical, and sexual abuse than cisgender people. Sexual abuse histories in childhood are not rare – usually because the child was gender atypical, was ostracised for that, and so was marked as vulnerable by the abuser. This, alongside adult gender dysphoria, can derange coping strategies to the degree that a Borderline Personality Disorder (BPD)/Emotionally Unstable Personality Disorder (EUPD)/Complex Post-Traumatic Stress Disorder (C-PTSD) diagnosis pertains. Fortunately, there is very often a gratifying reduction in the behaviours that lead to such a diagnosis when gender dysphoria is adequately addressed, not least because a significant stressor (and attendant maladaptive coping strategies) has been removed.

Of course, in a proportion of individuals who have attracted this diagnosis, it is perfectly reasonably made. We should note here, however, that gender is not cited as an aspect of identity disturbance in the ICD 11 diagnosis of 6D11.5 *Personality Disorder – Borderline Pattern,* as thinking has evolved from the ICD 10 diagnosis. We can therefore usually discount gender diversity in considering such diagnoses. Indeed the difficult thoughts, affect, and behaviours which attract the diagnosis often persist even though gender dysphoria is addressed. Usually though – again due to the removal of a major stressor – the manifestations of the condition are rather less marked and show the additional characteristic reduction from early middle life onwards that is so often seen. It is exceedingly uncommon for the manifestation of a personality disorder to grow worse when gender dysphoria is addressed, and this should accordingly prompt diagnostic review.

Body Dysmorphic Disorder (BDD)

Body dysmorphic disorder (BDD) is uncommon, but it can both intersect with and be a differential for gender dysphoria. Let us take the differential first. This usually occurs when a person has a pathological dislike of a gendered body part – most commonly the genitals or chest. The patient will almost invariably wish to remove the body part surgically, as there is a sense that the body part does not belong to them. This can, superficially, look like the trans or non-binary person's wish to have surgery; however, there are significant differences. In the case of the trans person, surgery is an act of creation – albeit via removal. It is as if one wishes to create a local park by removing the burnt-out cars, needles, and old mattresses and then planting a lawn and some flowers – removal as creation. The trans-masculine person wants a male chest – the removal of the breast tissue is incidental; the trans woman wants female genitalia – the removal of the penis is incidental. In contrast, the person with BDD of the chest simply wants it gone – and as a result often wishes to have a flat chest, with no nipples, shape, or anything else. Similarly, those with BDD of the genitals wish for simple removal rather than the creation of another set.[3] Further, those with BDD do not wish to actually be of another gender – they are quite happy as men, for example, but feel that their penis and/or testicles are not theirs – or may complain of chronic pain in the absence of any biological markers. Indeed, some people with BDD are very distressed and may endeavour to access gender services as a means of obtaining their desired treatments. Of course, this is not a gender matter, and diagnosis in these cases often serves to exclude gender dysphoria, rather than making any special claims about BDD treatments.

BDD can also occur in people with gender dysphoria. Cases where it relates to a lower limb, for example (which is rather more common than some other forms), need not detain us here, but it is worth considering those forms which relate to gender. The most frequent of these is usually a pathological dislike of facial features. Many trans people do dislike their facial features because they are usually uncovered, play such an important part in everyday interaction, and are markedly gendered. Facial surgery is therefore not uncommon, especially among trans women. The point of pathology is when it becomes an obsession or unreasonable to the everyday observer. For example, a patient may spend six or seven hours every day considering their face in the mirror or may refuse to leave the house or even their bedroom, for fear of how their face looks. In such instances, surgery is ineffective as the pathological cognition simply moves to another feature or the surgery is considered inadequate. The jaw which was too wide is still so and must therefore be operated on again, or it is now the nose which is abhorrent. This is quite different, of course, from the functional patient living an ordinary life, who, for reasons of function or aesthetics, wishes to alter their appearance.

Malingering

Aside from psychosis and BDD, there are very few occasions when another illness or disorder presents as gender dysphoria, and they have been detailed here and in Chapter 2, *Assessment*. It remains here to consider malingering: it bears repeating that gender dysphoria is not, in itself, a mental disorder but may perhaps be best seen as a part of human diversity and living which nonetheless brings with it a common need for medical assistance – as pregnancy does. It follows therefore that gender dysphoria alone is not a disability and does not preclude one from working or generally living life. However, difficulties can be associated with it, and these are particularly marked if there are intersections of marginalisation. A healthy, wealthy, well-supported, white person who can access medical care will very often do fine; a poor, unsupported, black person with a chronic illness who cannot access trans-related care is vastly less likely to be OK – and should be supported accordingly, ideally taking into account all their varying needs and intersections of identity.

Both these people are trans, of course, but just occasionally one comes across people who are not, but purport to be for secondary gain – the most common being in forensic settings (see Chapter 6, *Forensic Settings*). Malingering in such cases is often best identified by a gender identity clinic consultant psychiatrist or consultant psychologist who will wish to establish a robust history, diagnosis, and formulation.

---

[3] A small subset of gender-neutral people also wish for these things; however, discriminating from BDD and other conditions in these instances is extremely complex and should be undertaken by a gender identity clinic consultant psychiatrist or consultant psychologist.

Surgery in the Context of Serious, Chronic Psychiatric Illness

Notwithstanding those people considered earlier who are not trans and will therefore not have surgery, those trans people who wish to have surgeries need to be in the best possible shape beforehand, no matter what the surgery is related to. As a general principle, any health condition which can be optimised before surgery is undertaken, should be. This principle applies just as much to mental health as it does to physical health, of course. Patients who are actively psychotic, severely depressed, or manic are unable to cooperate properly with essential surgical aftercare instructions and will fare less well as a result. Most trans folk with a chronic mental illness diagnosis are aware of it or will readily accept it if they are not. It is important that they know that if their mental health is not as good as it can be when surgery is due, they should openly and honestly say so, confident that the surgery will be delayed to no greater extent than that necessary for them to regain equilibrium. Except in the most exceptional of cases, it is not appropriate for surgery to be refused or indefinitely delayed simply because the person just *might* become unwell in the course of a surgical admission.

Summary

In considering gender identity in the context of mental illness, it is striking how often it remains stable when so very much else of the person's life is affected by the illness. To some extent, this speaks to the heart of how innate gender and so trans identities are. This is not to say that if there is flux in the person's feelings about gender that treatment would be precluded, but that there would need to be a stable period of gender beforehand – a process of establishing what is right, especially in the context of a mental health difficulty, is entirely to be expected.

Consequently, treatment is by no means precluded for people with mental or physical health problems – but does need to be in a period of general stability and will invariably need to be a multidisciplinary collaboration between the team managing the patient, the gender clinic, and naturally the patient themself.

Further Reading

Richards, C., Bouman, W. P., & Barker, M. J. (eds.). (2018). *Genderqueer and non-binary genders*. London: Palgrave-Macmillan.

World Health Organization. (2019). *International statistical classification of diseases and related health problems 11*. Geneva: WHO.

References

Colizzi, M., Costa, R., & Todarello, O. (2014). Transsexual patients' psychiatric comorbidity and positive effect of cross-sex hormonal treatment on mental health: Results from a longitudinal study. *Psychoneuroendocrinology, 39*(1), 65–73.

Hill, D. B., Rozanski, C., Carfagnini, J., & Willoughby, B. (2005). Gender identity disorders in childhood and adolescence: A critical inquiry. In D. Karasic & J. Drescher (eds.), *Sexual and gender diagnoses of the diagnostic and statistical manual (DSM)* (pp. 7–34). New York: The Haworth Press.

Hoshiai, M., Matsumoto, Y., Sato, T., Ohnishi, M., Okabe, N., Kishimoto, Y., Terada, S., & Kuroda, S. (2010). Psychiatric comorbidity among patients with gender identity disorder. *Psychiatry and Clinical Neurosciences, 64*, 514–519.

Øien, R. A., Cicchetti, D. V., & Nordahl-Hansen, A. (2018). Gender dysphoria, sexuality and autism spectrum disorders: A systematic map review. *Journal of Autism and Developmental Disorders, 48* (12), 4028–4037.

Robles, R., Fresán, A., Vega-Ramírez, H., Cruz-Islas, J., Rodríguez-Pérez, V., Domínguez-Martínez, T., & Reed, G. M. (2016). Removing transgender identity from the classification of mental disorders: A Mexican field study for ICD-11. *The Lancet Psychiatry*, 3(9), 850–859.

Simon, L., Zsolt, U., Fogd, D., & Czobor, P. (2011). Dysfunctional core beliefs, perceived parenting behavior and psychopathology in gender identity disorder: A comparison of male-to-female, female-to-male transsexual and nontranssexual control subjects. *Journal of Behavior Therapy and Experimental Psychiatry 42*(1), 38–45.

World Health Organization. (1992). *International classification of diseases 10* (2nd ed.). Geneva: WHO.

(2019a). *ICD11: Classifying disease to map the way we live and die.* Retrieved 16 May 2019 from www.who.int/health-topics/international-classification-of-diseases

(2019b). *International statistical classification of diseases and related health problems 11.* Geneva: WHO.

Supporting Trans and Non-binary People in Mental Health Services

Chapter 5

Introduction

When faced with the significant personal difficulties patients presenting to mental health services bring, it is understandable that clinicians hesitate to manage gender as well – the need appears neither so necessary nor so immediate given the limited resources one has to draw upon. Harm management and capacity are naturally the primary considerations in such instances. Nonetheless due consideration must be given to a person's gender, just as we do with cisgender men and women – indeed, for trans people, matters of gender may be more pressing and therefore more pertinent to the clinical encounter than they are for cisgender people. For example, endeavouring to create a therapeutic alliance with a severely depressed individual to manage suicidal risk will be next to impossible if they are mis-gendered – that is, if they are referred to by an inappropriate name and pronouns. In this instance, to say that one is focusing on suicidality is to miss the point. Indeed, such an approach would only exacerbate the problem if the patient has a depressive illness pre-cipitated by their belief that they will not be accepted because of their trans status. This is not to say, of course, that one must immediately initiate cross-sex hormones in such instances, but that a holistic approach which includes gender (perhaps indicating facilitation of gender identity assessment for hormones upon recovery) will likely pay dividends.

Conversely, however, clinicians must be wary of diagnostic overshadowing where staff pay undue attention to the client's gender status to the exclusion of the presenting psychia-tric concern. This can sometimes occur because staff are so concerned to be seen *doing the right thing* that they forget the fundamental reason the person is in contact with services in the first place. While due dignity and respect must always be afforded to people's gender status, if they are seen for a psychotic illness, that should be the focus of the work. As ever, a balance of clinical priorities must be made with the client's health being paramount and the route to that health including accommodation and respect for their gender status.

Adult Mental Health Services – Outpatient

When seeing trans and non-binary people in an outpatient clinic, it is important to bear in mind that there is a long history of psychiatrists, psychologists, and other mental health professionals treating trans and non-binary people rather poorly. There is now a *Memorandum of Understanding* signed by the United Kingdom's Royal College of Psychiatrists and the British Psychological Society, along with many other organisations, which bans conversion 'therapies' (MoU, 2017); however, this was not always the case with such things as aversion 'therapies' including shock and emetics (Gelder & Marks, 1969), token economies (Mukaddes, 2002), and talking 'cures' (Turban et al., 2019) all having been tried in the past. Aside from the immorality of such approaches (which, of course, echoes those which tried to 'cure' non-heterosexual people), they simply do not work. Along with the pathologisation of gender diversity mentioned in the Introduction to this book, these historic treatment approaches have left those of us in the psychiatric and psychological professions in the rather unenviable position of quite often being prejudged by our clients as being opposed to gender diversity. Of course, psychiatrists, psychologists, and others take a variety of views from the affirmative to the un-affirming (and that is quite aside from those of us who are gender diverse ourselves); however, it is incumbent upon us as professionals to follow the current science and practice of our profession – which is unequivocally affirming of gender diversity in principle (BPS, 2019; RCPsych, 2013).

This historic opposition of the psychological professions to gender diversity, and associated prejudgement of them by clients, can unfortunately adversely colour the clinical encounter prior to its start. For this reason, it is important to consider the engagement of the client with the service prior to their actually sitting in the room with you. For example, if there is a questionnaire with only male or female tick boxes to be filled out by the client before seeing you, then that will exclude non-binary people as well as some trans people considering transition. Similarly, toilets only signed for males and females will exclude certain groups (we will consider inpatient facilities later). A receptionist calling loudly for "Mr Doe!" will upset Ms Doe if she is in female role.[1] It is relatively simple to mitigate this – a postcard size rainbow flag sticker on the front door is reassuring;[2] having an open text box for gender (and sexuality) on forms – and not ordering lists on such forms with Male, White, Married, and Heterosexual at the top; having a variety of magazines, including ones for gay and lesbian people; ensuring that images on posters and flyers are diverse; and ensuring adequate non-clinical as well as clinical staff training, all will create an impression of inclusion before the clinical encounter starts – and will make the clinical encounter itself much easier.

We have discussed in the Introduction how gender diversity is no longer considered pathological in its own right. There can be a tendency, however, to consider such a striking facet of a person's identity as necessarily a part of a presenting psychiatric issue. However, this risks misdiagnosis and an incorrect formulation. In the vast majority of cases, a person's gender status will not be a part of their psychopathology. Patients are significantly more likely to have an Emotionally Unstable Personality Disorder (EUPD)/Complex PTSD *and* be trans or non-binary – rather than their gender diversity likely part of their EUPD/Complex PTSD. Similarly, many people with an autistic spectrum condition are also trans or non-binary (see Chapter 7, *Autistic Spectrum Conditions and Intellectual Disability*; Glidden et al., 2016) – autistic perseverative special interest is very seldom a differential for gender diverse identities. While Ockham's Razor is a useful heuristic, we should be careful of an overly Procrustean reduction of human diversity – people are very often more than one thing at a time.

Trans and non-binary people have mental illnesses at approximately the same rate as the general population, including psychotic illnesses. There are higher rates of anxiety,

---

[1] An elegant solution to this is to use initial and surname – calling for "J Doe" makes no assumption of gender. Of course, this must be for all patients so as not to focus on the trans patient.

[2] Staff must know what it means, of course. For those unfamiliar, it is the universal symbol of lesbian, gay, bisexual, and transgender (as well as other forms of gender and sexual diversity) pride and inclusion.

depression, and self-harm due to minority or marginalisation stress –the stress of being part of a group which is subject to prejudice – but these return to roughly population rates when trans people's identity is accepted (Robles et al., 2016). This is not to say that being trans does not inflect a patient's experience of their condition or illness – just as occurs with any other demographic such as race, ethnicity, religion, and so on – it is simply that it is not causal. For example, a trans person may be wise to be cautious of certain situations for fear of physical violence; this will naturally inflect their psychopathological paranoia. The art is in not only accepting that they will inevitably be under scrutiny or attack (they will not) but also in not disavowing their lived experience (trans people are more at risk than cisgender people).

On the rare occasions when it genuinely does appear that the patient's illness or condition is presenting as gender dysphoria, then a second opinion from a gender identity clinic consultant psychiatrist or consultant psychologist would be a wise consideration. For reasons stated earlier, misattributing gender diversity to pathology could lead to misdiagnosis, may irreparably damage therapeutic rapport, and indeed may cause significant decompensation. If we recall the diathesis-stress model of mental distress, we can see that one may have a predisposition towards a certain illness, whether through genetics, circumstance, or both; in addition, under increased stress, decompensation is increasingly likely. Thus, misgendering and managing a trans identity in an unsupportive environment is such a cause of stress for trans people as to make decompensation under these circumstances almost inevitable. Ironically, this can be attributed by clinicians (who are perhaps overloaded and not paying sufficient attention) to the trans status itself or to the trans behaviours exacerbating the illness and so being further repressed by staff – and thus causing more stress – in a vicious circle. Conversely, those clinicians who are supportive of a trans identity or the exploration of that identity will likely form better rapport and so have much more chance of a beneficial clinical encounter.

Even a simple referral to a gender identity clinic can take the stress out of the situation and lead to better rapport. It goes without saying that such referral should never be as a 'reward' for treatment compliance, any more than referral for any other medical condition would be. We would not, for example, only refer a patient to a diabetologist upon condition of psychiatric treatment compliance. For clarity, the usual diagnosis which pertains here is *Gender Incongruence* (ICD 11), for more information on this see the Introduction.

That said, *treatment* (in contrast to assessment) by a gender identity clinic is likely to be predicated upon a person's mental illness being well managed – for the simple reason that the patient will need to consent, to arrive in a timely manner for review, to take their medicine regularly, to have regular blood tests, and to manage the psychological adaptations precipitated by cross-sex hormones and/or surgeries, for example (WPATH, 2011; forthcoming 2020). Treatment recommendations from gender identity clinics are therefore made in close concert with the person's mental health team. This naturally becomes more complex if a patient is in an inpatient setting, especially if they are likely to remain so for a significant period of time; therefore, it is to this which we now turn.

Adult Mental Health Services – Inpatient

If a person is so unwell as to require acute inpatient psychiatric care (care for chronic conditions is another matter), it would be unusual for assessment or treatment for gender dysphoria to start at that point, although it would be quite reasonable to refer during this period for an assessment upon discharge from the inpatient unit. (Treatment already initiated should, of course, be continued just as with treatment for any other medical condition.) It is, however, not uncommon for trans people to decide to act upon their feelings when encountering a major life event – and a psychiatric hospitalisation may be just such an instance. A closeted trans person who has endeavoured to take their own life and is hospitalised, for example, may decide that "enough is enough" and that to come out is a better option than living miserably.[3] In this instance, managing their gender is vital to treatment for their admitting condition and should be facilitated. Even when a person is admitted for another matter such as psychosis and then comes out about their gender there is benefit in managing both the illness and the gender dysphoria as we have seen earlier. Indeed, aside from equalities law, if the person is held under the Mental Health Act, not to accommodate their gender could unnecessarily increase the length of their detention, the legality of which could then be called into question.

The matter is a little more complicated for people with more chronic disorders who may be in secure conditions for many months or years. In this instance, referral for assessment by consultant psychiatrists and consultant psychologists at a gender identity clinic should be undertaken so that a collaborative approach may be arrived at by all parties. There is sometimes a fear that clinicians at gender identity clinics will always immediately treat upon referral. This is not the case. A referral is always for *assessment* – treatment is a quite separate matter. However, it should be borne in mind that after substantial appropriate assessment, treatment with cross-sex hormones or surgeries *may* be a legitimate aim for a recognised diagnosis, and facilitating this in the inpatient setting may be beneficial for both the patient and the treating staff.

Single-sex Facilities

It goes without saying that if a person is admitted who has already transitioned to another gender, then no attempt to de-transition them should be made. This would be grossly unethical and indeed could lead to significant suicidal risk. Hormonal treatment should be maintained and their preferred name should be used, as should their preferred clothing. The trans person may need assistance with self-care if unwell, as with any other patient, and this should include trans-specific care. For example, facial hair removal for trans women will be vital, leaving facial hair to grow as with a cisgender male is unacceptable. Similarly, they may need help with dilation – the placing of an acrylic stent in the neo-vagina every few days for 20 minutes or so; there are health implications if this is not done, including frequent infection of the stenosed vagina and concomitant urinary tract infections. Healthcare staff who are able to deal with colostomy bags and tampons in the ordinary course of their work should have no difficulties with patient care such as this.

A further consideration is that some trans people have been disowned by their genetic relations and may have a *family of choice* – sometimes rather pleasingly called a *framily*. Due consideration should be given as to where support or stress is to be found, as good social support is consistently linked with reducing self-harm and suicidality among trans people. Genetic relatives may claim privilege on that basis alone but may be a cause of distress and, as ever, assumptions in this regard may need further investigation. In addition, some trans people may find links with LGBT+ groups extremely helpful. This could be facilitated by

---

[3] It almost invariably is.

staff through arranging in-reach by these organisations, although trans people should not be assumed to be part of an LGBT+ 'community' any more than one would assume someone from an ethnic minority background would necessarily attend a community group based on that characteristic.

Mental health staff are, on the whole, extremely skilled, compassionate, and supportive. However, some can raise objections to gender diversity, most commonly through unfamiliarity, although sometimes through religious or cultural beliefs. Those who object should be reminded of their obligation to the organisation and profession rather than their personal wishes. Similarly 'jokes', misgendering, and so on should be made clear as unacceptable by staff or patients.

There is sometimes a question of other patients objecting, but as being trans is perfectly legal – indeed is legally protected by the Gender Recognition Act 2004 and the Single Equality Act 2010 – there is no right to object. It can sometimes be helpful to substitute another demographic characteristic such as ethnicity as a thought experiment – how would we respond if patients or staff objected to having someone of a particular ethnicity on the ward? Concerns can arise around sexualised behaviour, but they are no more likely among trans people than cisgender people. If concerns occur, they should be dealt with as psychopathology or as a criminal matter, as appropriate, just as with cisgender people, but they have nothing to do with trans status. Training on all of these concerns is available and should be sought out, as should training on gender diversity generally – it is not reasonable to ask a patient who is unwell to provide free continuing professional development. Psychiatrists and psychologists are ideally placed to take leadership roles in engendering a culture of affirmation and acceptance,[4] as when staff are reassured there is often rather less of an issue than was initially feared.

A person who has transitioned should be accommodated with people of the same gender – that is, trans women should be with cisgender women, and trans men should be with cisgender men. Staff of the same gender should undertake intimate searches. Where a person has just come out about their gender, or if they are non-binary, flexible solutions should be sought – if at all possible in concert with the patient. For example, a side room may be used or night accommodation may be in one place with day accommodation in another. This should only be an interim measure until more satisfactory solutions can be found. The dignity and privacy of the trans or non-binary person should be respected at all times and should not come second to expediency. Simply defaulting to birth-assigned sex is unacceptable.

Searching

Searching is often a difficult matter when a person has not transitioned. We should note that a person may have fully transitioned, indeed may have legally changed gender in the United Kingdom without having surgery or hormones of any kind. Someone of the same gender should search a person who has fully transitioned. The police have the elegant solution of asking staff of the same gender to search a person who has not fully transitioned, but the staff member has a right to decline and another staff member may be found. The staff member declining may require further training.

---

[4] Not 'tolerance', no-one wants to be 'tolerated': it implies the person is doing something untoward when they are not.

Gender Recognition Act

We should note that in the United Kingdom, there is no requirement for a person to have a new birth certificate or a Gender Recognition Certificate to be treated as their identified gender. To be protected under law, one merely has to be "intending to undergo gender reassignment" – note the *intending*. No certificates of physical treatments are required. It is not acceptable, ethical, or in many cases legal to require people to provide paperwork to 'prove' their gender. Please see Chapter 9, *Legal and Religious Aspects* for more information on the law, including around the legal situation pertaining to disclosure of a person's trans status.

Summary

Trans people will access mental health services for the same range of reasons cisgender people do. Their mental health problems may be exacerbated by prejudice or by not being treated as their experienced gender; efforts to mitigate stressors such as these are likely to benefit treatment for the presenting concern. Mitigating stressors in this way can require a culture change and psychiatrists and psychologists, usually being senior members of staff, are well placed to effect such culture change.

Further Reading

British Psychological Society. (2019). *Guidelines for psychologists working with gender, sexuality and relationship diversity* (2nd ed.). London: British Psychological Society.

Royal College of Nursing. (2016). *Fair care for trans people: A RCN guide for nursing and healthcare professionals*. London: Royal College of Nursing.

Royal College of Psychiatrists. (2013). *CR181 Good practice guidelines for the assessment and treatment of gender dysphoria*. London: Royal College of Psychiatrists.

World Professional Association for Transgender Health (WPATH) (forthcoming 2020). *Standards of care for transgender and gender non-conforming people Version 8*. Illinois: WPATH.

References

British Psychological Society. (2019). *Guidelines for psychologists working with gender, sexuality and relationship diversity* (2nd ed.). London: British Psychological Society.

Gelder, M. G., & Marks, I. M. (1969). Aversion treatment in transvestism and transsexualism. In R. Green & J. Money (eds.), *Transsexualism and sex reassignment* (pp. 383–413). Baltimore: The Johns Hopkins UniversityPress.

Glidden, D., Bouman, W. P., Jones, B. A., & Arcelus, J. (2016). Gender dysphoria and autism spectrum disorder: A systematic review of the literature. *Sexual Medicine Reviews, 4*(1), 3–14.

Memorandum of Understanding on Conversion Therapy in the UK Version 2. (2017). Retrieved 16 February 2018 from www.pinktherapy.com/portals/0/MoU2_Final.pdf

Mukaddes, N. M. (2002). Gender identity problems in autistic children. *Child: Care, Health and Development, 28*, 529–532.

Robles, R., Fresán, A., Vega-Ramírez, H., Cruz-Islas, J., Rodríguez-Pérez, V., Domínguez-Martínez, T., & Reed, G. M. (2016). Removing transgender identity from the classification of mental disorders: a Mexican field study for ICD-11. *The Lancet Psychiatry, 3*(9), 850–859.

Royal College of Psychiatrists. (2013). *CR181 Good practice guidelines for the assessment and treatment of gender dysphoria*. London: Royal College of Psychiatrists.

Turban J. L., Beckwith, N., Reisner, S. L., & Keuroghlian, A. S. (2019). Association between recalled exposure to gender identity conversion efforts and psychological distress and suicide attempts among transgender adults. *JAMA Psychiatry.* doi:10.1001/jamapsychiatry.2019.2285

World Professional Association for Transgender Health (WPATH) (2011). *Standards of care for transgender and gender non-conforming people Version 7.* Illinois: WPATH.

(forthcoming 2020). *Standards of care for transgender and gender non-conforming people Version 8.* Illinois: WPATH.

Supporting Trans and Non-binary People in Forensic Settings

Introduction

Criminal offending is not the norm and gender dysphoria is comparatively rare. The combination of the two, accordingly, is so infrequent that there is little published literature, and none of it even attempts statistical validity. In this specialised element of an already specialised field within a medical specialism, any learning must inevitably, perhaps, be experiential. Experience grows patient by patient, and knowledge and judgement correspondingly improve. It is for this reason that trans folk in forensic settings present the greatest challenges and require every ounce of multidisciplinary attention that can be afforded. This chapter does not specifically cover trans people in the secure estate who have an autistic condition or an intellectual disability (see Chapter 7, *Autistic Spectrum Conditions and Intellectual Disability*); however, the principles outlined here may apply also for those who have been diverted into the mental health system, or who are in the secure mental health estate as discussed later.

Trans Folk as Victims of Crime

Sadly, trans folk are usually involved in forensic matters solely in the role of victim, perhaps especially if they have another intersecting form of marginalisation such as mental health problems, ethnicity, religion, an autistic spectrum condition, and so on. Whilst they might be no more likely to be a victim than anyone else for many crimes, (burglary, for example), often they are subject to crimes motivated by the personal dislike of others. Assaults, verbal, physical, and sometimes sexual in nature, are encountered and are much like those experienced by gay men in past decades. These crimes are related to the obviously trans status of the victim and sadly are all too often underpinned by an exploitative and unhelpful media that seeks to sell copy through the vilification of the minority group du jour.

The detection of previously unsuspected trans status may sometimes precipitate assault, particularly if that detection occurs in a sexual context, consensual or otherwise. The police are now particularly skilled at dealing with sexual assaults and crimes motivated by prejudice, and trans people very often report a satisfactory policing response. Unfortunately, this has not always been so; many trans people have been subject to anti-LGBT policing strategies in the past. For this reason, trans people may be wary of police contact and may need support to report crimes so that the perpetrator is prevented from victimising others.

Whilst being identifiable as a trans person can cause the problems described here, it should be noted that achieving a change of gender role where no one is aware of the person's trans status (sometimes termed 'stealth' or 'going stealth') also carries with it vulnerabilities, particularly to blackmail. Indeed, there have tragically been deaths by suicide of trans people who have been blackmailed and [wrongly] believed the police would not be receptive and that anyone knowing their trans status would be intolerable.

Trans Folk as Both Offenders and Victims

Sometimes trans folk are involved in crime, in whatever capacity, because they are trans; sometimes their trans status is unrelated to their offending but affects how they are treated by the justice system. Further, trans folk may be convicted in circumstances that do not seem entirely fair in that someone born into their gender role would, one imagines, not have been accused or prosecuted or, if convicted, would have attracted a lesser penalty. Trans folk can seem to be both perpetrator and, in another sense, victim. One example occurs when a person who has engaged in a sexual relationship with a trans person seeks to bring charges on grounds of deception purely because the person is trans and the person claims ignorance of that fact. Sadly, convictions have been made on this basis. One wonders whether such convictions, or even charges, would have been made if someone did not disclose ethnic heritage, for example, and was accused of deception.

Trans People Who Are Offenders

Aside from being victims of crime, or being involved in crime 'because' they are trans, some trans people offend for reasons which are indeed related to their gender or transition – for example, stealing make-up or clothing because it is "too embarrassing" to buy it and then being arrested and convicted for shoplifting, committing assault on a person engaging in transphobic abuse, taking illicit drugs to manage gender dysphoria, or (especially in countries without nationalised healthcare) stealing or engaging in criminal activities to fund physical treatments such as hormones or surgeries. In these instances, trans-related healthcare while in the justice system can pay dividends, as gender issues may be part of the root of the offending behaviour. Indeed, if a person is able to work on accepting their trans status in therapy, they may not feel the need to steal make-up. If they can gain hormones through the NHS or a not-for-profit provider, they may not need to finance them through criminal activity.

Nonetheless, the faulty [criminal] problem-solving must be addressed as part of the treatment for offending. This may include work in the secure estate; with probation, and/or with LGBT support groups either via in-reach or in the community; or work on arousal and management of the threat response which can accompany being trans.

One matter of pertinence to be considered here is that of sex work. Some trans people, perhaps especially trans women, find that sex work not only provides an income with which to fund treatments but also may provide an apparently supportive community. Again, this is perhaps especially the case in countries without nationalised healthcare, but it is not unheard of in the United Kingdom. Specific support and advice may be needed in such cases – where the offender is also a victim and faces further marginalisation by virtue of their trans status.

Offenders Purporting to Be Trans

The same arguments seen earlier that offending is related to being trans can sometimes be made [fallaciously] by sex offenders who assert that they were abusing children or adults as part of their 'exploration' of gender. This is, of course, almost invariably false, as the vast majority of people explore gender roles in adolescence and childhood and do not commit deviant sexual acts while doing so. Further, trans and non-binary adults do not commit sexual offences as part of their exploration of gender – the very idea would be abhorrent. The assertion therefore that sexual abuse is a part of being trans is incorrect and is likely an attempted abrogation of responsibility on the part of the abuser. Similarly, some people with very lengthy sentences for violent crime may seek to have them reduced through claiming that the offence was precipitated by their being trans, or that as they are now female (these arguments are seldom made by trans men or non-binary people), they are a lower risk. Indeed, it is striking that it is almost unheard of for an ordinary trans person to commit a serious sexual offence after transition, whereas sexual offenders do purport to be trans after offending. Again this is not to say that sexual offenders who transition will therefore be of lower risk (no evidence shows that they will), as this group is, necessarily, markedly different from trans people who have not offended.

For this reason, whilst in ordinary practice one would rightly take a trans person at their word, in the case of offenders, especially sexual offenders, this often cannot be assumed. Aside from seeking release or abrogation of responsibility, people already in the secure estate for a protracted period for reasons connected with sexual or other deviant behaviour may make the claim that they are trans for secondary gain. This may include such things as seeking to be in the same part of the secure estate as family members or others with whom they have strong connections (sometimes co-defendants), having a closer proximity to potential victims, sexual gratification elicited by being treated as an intimate confidante by women, acquiring some sort of 'special' status, or the requirement for the person to adopt an ever more female role by an offender partner.

The secure estate is unpleasant and boring but offers unique opportunities for networking with others. Offenders will, perhaps understandably, do a great deal to make their lot even slightly better and have a very great deal of time to devote to thinking of ways of achieving this. Status within an incarcerated community is a major determinant of quality of life, and those offenders who are low on the social pecking order (perhaps by virtue of a sexual crime) may discover that the penal system is [rightly] obliged to accommodate and support gender diversity. For example, separate showering facilities must be provided, searching must be discreet and take due account of gender, and separate laundry facilities may be provided. All this can be decidedly attractive in an environment where one would otherwise be indistinguishable from the surrounding multitude. Accordingly, the motivation behind such requests merits extremely careful consideration, usually over the course of multiple assessments and with much discussion among the assessing clinicians. It can be especially useful therefore if the assessing clinicians are highly experienced and come from slightly different professional backgrounds – one useful model is having a consultant psychologist in gender, a consultant psychiatrist in gender, and a non-gender specialist consultant forensic psychologist or psychiatrist who all assess together. Some clinicians are concerned that consultants working in gender will be unduly relaxed in recommending treatments, but this is not so. Almost invariably, they will have worked in other settings, and will also have extensive experience in the field. Treatments are most assuredly not guaranteed – assiduous assessment is.

The Choice of Gendered Estate

Trans folk arrested for, or convicted of, offences which are usually unrelated to their gender attract particular attention about place of confinement because it is sometimes unclear whether the offender should be sent to a men's or a women's facility. Defence counsel may argue that a custodial sentence would be particularly harsh in view of their client's circumstances and may suggest that a non-custodial penalty would be appropriate. The impression is that this argument is fairly often accepted.

If a custodial sentence is awarded, it used to be that the destination estate entirely hinged on whether or not the detained person possessed a Gender Recognition Certificate; all other factors and circumstances were ignored. Unfortunately, many genuinely trans offenders had been living for a significant period of time in their gender but were illiterate, too poor, or otherwise too chaotic to undergo the fairly costly and bureaucratic process required to gain a Gender Recognition Certificate. This policy therefore distressingly often gave rise to wholly unsatisfactory placements in which trans offenders were vulnerable to assault, ridicule, and unwanted sexual attention – with tragic suicides sometimes being the result.

A more recent change in policy has thankfully brought in a more nuanced approach whereby offenders claiming trans status in the absence of any supporting documentation are considered by a specially convened Transgender Case Board (see National Offender Management Service, 2017; NHS England, 2018) and allocated to one of five distinct categories:

1. Those offenders with a Gender Recognition Certificate, who must be placed in the estate denoted by that certificate, and treatment continued.
2. Those trans offenders whose change of social gender role seems to have been well established for some time (usually before commission of the offence). Often they are already taking hormone treatment and may have had some surgical interventions. Such offenders should be placed in the estate consistent with their social gender role, with treatment continued, unless there is an extraordinary reason to do otherwise.
3. Offenders whose change of gender role is equivocal, partial, intermittent, or otherwise questionable. The destination estate could be either the male or the female estate, depending on those particular, individual circumstances, with the preference of the offender being a factor to consider with all the others, of course. It may be that further establishment of role while in the secure estate leads to a subsequent move to the estate of the other gender. Consideration should be given to an assessment by a Gender Identity Clinic psychiatrist or Gender Identity Clinic psychologist.
4. Offenders with very little to support the claim of trans status other than the statement of the offender in question. In this case, the estate is usually that consistent with sex assigned at birth, with consideration of an assessment from a Gender Identity Clinic psychiatrist or Gender Identity Clinic psychologist.
5. The last category is that it is strongly suspected that a malicious or dishonest claim of trans status is being made (see earlier section). Such suspicions may come from the secure estate intelligence sources, statements from other offenders, or intercepted communication from the offender. Again, the estate is that consistent with sex assigned at birth, with consideration of an assessment from a Gender Identity Clinic psychiatrist or Gender Identity Clinic psychologist, who should be fully informed of those suspicions.

All trans offenders seem to be treated as 'vulnerable offenders' or placed in a medical wing – at least at first. Later, if things go well, they may be moved to ordinary offender status. The vulnerability of the trans offender seems to be linked to the disposition of the offender and the robust anti-bullying and integration policies in place in the institution. Such a move can also be useful for the purposes of assessment by a Gender Identity Clinic psychiatrist or Gender Identity Clinic psychologist.

Incarcerated People Newly Asserting Trans Status

People already in the secure estate who claim trans status present two major problems. The first is that of the diagnosis, formulation, and treatment plan. The second is the challenge of providing gender-related treatment to an incarcerated person.

Upon entry into the secure estate, some people immediately declare that they are trans in the absence of any previous declaration on the 'outside'. While this should be viewed with *some* suspicion (see later), we should be cognisant that the person has seen the entire structure of their life collapse – for example, their mortgage or rent will go unpaid, and they will lose their accommodation. Any standing they had in their social circle is utterly gone. Their source of income entirely ceases. Life will never, ever, be the same again. If part of that life was keeping a tenacious grip on gender conformity in the face of ever-growing gender dysphoria, the brakes are abruptly removed, so to speak. With nothing left to lose, they may as well be hung for a sheep as a lamb and just admit their long-concealed trans status. In such cases, a swift review by a gender identity clinic psychiatrist or gender identity clinic psychologist will pay dividends as at least something will be being sorted out – one small step on the road to a better life.

Nevertheless, it can be a matter of concern if offenders report a trans identity seemingly out of the blue – and especially after some time in the secure estate. Claims of long-standing cross-gender identification with both childhood and adulthood cross-dressing are often made in these circumstances. These claims are sometimes related in earlier psychiatric reports as if they are established facts when, on closer examination, they are merely earlier renditions of the same assertion. Such claims or statements, by the offender or by earlier assessors, merit the very closest scrutiny and should only be accepted as definite biographical facts if there is some evidence for them other than simply the offender's assertion that they are true. An offender whose gender identity clearly pre-dates their offence is a lot less worrying than an offender who claims a lifelong gender dysphoria which, oddly, no one noticed at the time and which they entirely omitted to mention earlier.

Diagnosis

With regard to diagnosis, as we have seen earlier, it has sometimes naively been assumed that anyone declaring an aspiration to live in another social gender role will be doing so without any covert agenda and that therefore a diagnosis of *HA60 Gender Incongruence* applies – indeed all diagnostic classification is based on that assumption. While people at liberty are free to change their social gender role at any time and have far less secondary gain from malingering, people in the secure estate have more complex aetiologies and consequently diagnosis becomes more complex. One of the matters for clarification is how a person fares in their gender role – does it make them less dysphoric and more functional? The secure estate protocols currently act to accommodate this through the possible movement to the sex of identity, not birth – but whether this is a right or a privilege in all cases is unclear.

A further complicating factor is that the practical manifestation of gender reassignment, once under way, can be used to manipulate the penal system. Offenders may refuse to cooperate further or revert to their original gender role if their treatment does not progress in the manner they want or at a rate they would prefer. The administrative chaos that results can be ameliorated by acceding to their requests, but such accession simply serves to pile up problems for the future and reinforces the utility of such behaviour in the mind of the offender concerned.

Offenders claiming trans status may challenge the therapeutic elements of a custodial sentence, particularly treatment for sexual offending. Offenders may suggest that a change of gender role renders it an unnecessary reminder of an earlier, soon to be abandoned, male role. This is false because personality, personal history, and personal responsibility are continuous across anyone's lifespan – whatever their social gender role. Avoiding the treatment for sexual offending may, for some, even amount to a motive for claiming a trans identity. It might be more reasonably argued, though, that for trans offenders any treatment for sexual offending might be better delivered in an individual, one-to-one manner rather than in a group setting.

For clarity, some people endeavour to split themselves into a bad, violent, male part and a new 'gentle, non-violent, female' part. This is absolutely false (and indeed carries a misunderstanding of gender which rather brings into question the veracity of the purported unequivocal sense of gender identity). It is imperative that the person understands that, male, female, or non-binary, it was they who committed the offence for which they have been convicted. Further, the offender may think that they can convince others that they are less dangerous and therefore should be moved to a lower category of security with greater concomitant freedoms or indeed should be more likely to be granted parole. To be clear, while reducing the stressor of living in the wrong gender role may make a genuinely trans offender more amenable to treatment for offending, transitioning to a female role does not, in itself, reduce offending risk.

Indeed, many offenders, trans or otherwise, claim to have experienced a Damascene conversion to their true, female identity, or to God, or whatever else. Such claims are generally viewed with a sensible dose of scepticism but sometimes with a rather less healthy element of cynicism. Some Damascene conversions *do* occur, of course (Paul's did). Those conversions that endure long term seem to have been built on a solid foundation of the offender fully appreciating the horror of what was done and simply not wanting to be that person any more. A seeming conversion that doesn't involve a full acceptance of the earlier offences and appreciation of their nature – and the considerable psychological work that goes with this – will almost inevitably be shallow rooted or disingenuous.

Treatment

If there is an established diagnosis of *HA60 Gender Incongruence* that precedes incarceration, or if a diagnosis is firmly established after incarceration, it is still wise to work on the principle that reversible steps should have happened with demonstrable success before irreversible steps are considered. Generally, a change of social gender role should precede treatment with cross-sex hormones, and robust success in living in the new social gender role should precede irreversible surgery. The patient's hormonal milieu before surgery should, by means of hormones and, in people assigned male at birth, a gonadotrophin-releasing hormone analogue, be made the same as would be the case after that surgery.

There should, however, be caution around giving people in the secure estate personal access to medications which may cause harm to others, including testosterone gel. Instead, injections such as Sustanon or Nebido administered by healthcare providers could be considered. Similarly, it should be ensured that only the patient they are prescribed to takes the oestrogens. These are not reasons to withhold treatments, of course, any more than one would withhold treatment for any other diagnosed condition. Similarly, trans men or trans-masculine people may need access to tampons or sanitary towels, and post genital surgery trans women will need dilators, which are a matter of trans-related healthcare and must not be withheld.

The problem for those in the secure estate is that in virtually all cases, they will eventually be released back to ordinary society, albeit perhaps with parole conditions or on a life licence. It is unclear the extent to which living in a different gender role in the secure estate environment predicts living with similar success outside the secure estate because prisons can be surprisingly accommodating places. Offenders are obliged to live, long term, in close proximity to people they might otherwise cross the street to avoid. If they, or those they live with, act aggressively or violently, they incur immediate, practical penalties. Further, they have no responsibility to arrange accommodation, food supplies, heating, insurance, utilities, and the very many other things that constitute surviving outside the secure estate. Many offenders were notably maladroit at these aspects of living before their admission to the secure estate, and this may have been an active factor leading up to their incarceration.

Being accepted in a female role in a men's secure estate is one thing, but it does not necessarily predict managing in such a role in the female secure estate. Some offenders who were assigned male at birth harbour the happy delusion that women in an all-female social environment live a blissfully placid and cooperative lifestyle and cannot be disabused of this notion until transfer to a women's secure estate brings these false notions sharply to their attention. Further, in the male secure estate acceptance as a woman at eleven o'clock in the morning in the secure estate wing is not the same as acceptance as a woman at eleven o'clock at night on the local high street. Indeed, some feminine people report that their femininity was so marked in the hyper-masculine environment of a male wing as to make them sure they were women, when, upon release into the community with all its various expressions of gender, they thought they might be feminine men after all. It is hard to know how well offenders will cope with this social variation and lack of acceptance by others (sometimes with the threat of violence) unless they have experienced it in the real world. It is, however, vitally important to know how well they will cope because their response to such behaviour is sometimes the reason they were in the secure estate in the first place.

Accordingly, unless they are serving an extremely long or whole-life sentence, it does not seem sensible for offenders to undergo genital surgery unless they are spending at least a proportion of their time in a normal, civilian, social environment. Towards the end of sentences, offenders are usually moved to lower-category prisons, often with periods of leave, at first accompanied by an officer in civilian clothes, and later in an unaccompanied but regulated manner. Such leaves provide an opportunity to assess the extent to which a seemingly successful acceptance in a new social gender role will be maintained in the real, day-to-day, world.

Sometimes, offenders make the sensible decision not to embark upon any change of social gender role until they have been discharged from the secure estate on parole or a life licence. The change to a different social gender role may be particularly problematic for those offenders who are on a life licence because they may be terrified of provoking so negative a reaction from others that a public disturbance results and they are arrested in the ensuing fuss. They not unreasonably fear being returned to the secure estate and enduring a glacially slow investigation before their innocence can be established and their re-release secured.

Gender Recognition Certificates

There is no reason why an offender cannot apply for a Gender Recognition Certificate (GRC) in the United Kingdom and many have done so, although they cannot compel a clinician to provide reports for the Gender Recognition Panel. Indeed, the Gender Recognition Panel has awarded GRCs to people in the secure estate, and this triggers their immediate transfer to the estate devoted to their new, now legal, sex. Some offenders in this circumstance seem to cope very well (usually those with a clear history of gender dysphoria pre-dating incarceration), but for others (often those without such a history) the transfer is stormy.

It does not follow that the acquisition of a GRC renders the holder automatically eligible for physical treatments. Outside the provisions of the Mental Health Act and other circumstances where capacity is lacking, no doctor should advise or provide any treatment of any sort to anyone unless the patient gives informed consent and the doctor thinks that the treatment would be in the best interests of the patient. It is not possible for medical doctors or applied psychologists to be compelled to undertake or refer for treatments that they do not think are in their patients' interests, even if the patient insists upon this as a supposed right. Indeed, it does not follow that a person with a GRC will necessarily merit physical treatments because the law was written specifically to exclude physical treatments being a requirement (see Chapter 9, *Legal and Religious Aspects*). One does not have to have hormones or surgeries to obtain a GRC, as we recognise that these things are not necessarily constituent factors of one's gender. It reciprocally follows therefore that a person with a GRC will not in all cases wish to have physical treatments; therefore, a person who wishes to do so must be evaluated for each of these on a case-by-case basis.

Non-binary People

We have spoken here mostly about male and female people, rather than non-binary people, largely on the basis that the criminal justice system is, as yet, unaccommodating of non-binary identities. Within the law, one is male or female. Of course, this is neither biologically nor socially wholly the case (cf. Fausto-Sterling, 2012; Fine, 2011). Accommodating non-binary people is therefore rather challenging under the current system. All of the considerations detailed earlier should be considered, and due care should be given to consider the non-binary person's own views on where they should be best accommodated within the available options. It may be that special measures are necessary, as with other people from minority communities or those with special needs.

Secure Mental Health Services

Many of the considerations detailed here will also be appropriate for those people who have been diverted or transferred into secure mental health services (see Chapter 5, *Supporting Trans and Non-binary People in Mental Health Services*), although with the added complexity that some question of capacity will likely occur. Sadly, some of our colleagues in forensic mental health services can be tempted to elide gender dysphoria with whatever diagnosis underlies the reason for mental health involvement. Indeed, there can be a temptation to defer all treatment until after discharge from mental health services – whether to prison or the community. All of the considerations presented here regarding malingering apply – but a de facto assumption of the invalidity of a putative trans person's identity should not be made, not least because endeavouring to treat a trans person's mental disorder without accommodating their gender will almost invariably fail.

Summary

Trans people in the secure estate present a unique challenge for psychiatrists and psychologists, who must consider malingering alongside the very necessary treatment of gender dysphoria. As an added complexity, a lack of treatment of trans people for their gender dysphoria may prevent successful treatment of offending. Some treatment may be best undertaken in the secure estate, while some may need to wait until release. In almost all cases, obtaining an assessment from a consultant psychologist in gender, a consultant psychiatrist in gender, and a consultant forensic psychologist or psychiatrist, either at point of admission or when the person comes out about their gender, will be invaluable.

Further Reading

National Offender Management Service (NOMS). (2017). *The care and management of transgender offenders.* London: NOMS.

NHS England. (2018). *Interim guidance for the management of trans patients in adult secure services.* London: NHS England.

References

Fausto-Sterling, A. (2012). *Sex/gender: Biology in a social world.* London: Routledge.

Fine, C. (2011). *Delusions of gender: The real science behind sex differences.* London: Icon Books Ltd.

National Offender Management Service (NOMS). (2017). *The care and management of transgender offenders.* London: NOMS.

NHS England. (2018). *Interim guidance for the management of trans patients in adult secure services.* London: NHS England.

Autistic Spectrum Conditions and Intellectual Disability

Introduction

The autistic spectrum conditions, disorders, or diversity (ASC), which used to be known as Asperger's syndrome and autism, are in this chapter considered in tandem with intellectual disability (ID). While there are, of course, notable differences between the groups, we decided that for ease of reading, it was reasonable to consider all these conditions here. While we would not wish to elide them altogether, there has been some practical cross-over in some instances. It is notable that as the frequency of ASC diagnosis has risen, a proportionate decrease in diagnoses of mild ID has occurred. It's notable also that until quite recently, ASC was a purely paediatric diagnosis, with the assumption on the part of statutory care and other services that when children with Asperger's syndrome or autism passed the age of majority, they experienced an abrupt and overnight resolution. In fact, and totally unsurprisingly, children with ASC simply turn into adults with ASC, formally diagnosed or not. The only caveat is that trans boys – that is, those who are assigned female at birth but with a male identity – often like playing with mechanical toys, are less pro-social than their [cisgender] female peers, and can be socially isolated (because they seem like an 'odd' girl). They can look very much like a girl with ASC but are, in fact, typical of a [neurotypical, trans] boy.

In the population presenting to a UK National Health Service gender identity clinic (GIC), the rate of diagnosed ASC is about ten times that found in the general population at about 10%. There is a strong impression, also, that a fair few of the remaining 90% have some autistic spectrum traits. Currently, birth-assigned sex ratio at a GIC is about 1:1 of people assigned female at birth compared to those assigned male – it is worth noting here that ASC is a rarer diagnosis in cisgender females so the rate of ASC in trans men is vastly greater than that seen in the general population of those assigned female at birth (although, of course, it is closer to the gender of identity). Turning it round the other way, in a general population of adults diagnosed with ASC, it's remarkable how gender neutral the population is (and indeed what a high rate of non-heterosexuality is found therein).

It follows therefore that psychiatrists and psychologists who see people with ASC will likely come across some people who are also trans or, quite often, non-binary. While some cases of an autistic special interest are located towards gender, and the person thereby becomes confused (see later), in the vast majority of cases the person will indeed be trans or non-binary and should be treated accordingly. Naturally many people with ASC need no particular special assistance aside from some reasonable mannered accommodation such as we all might expect for all our various differences. In this instance, the ASC will naturally inflect the understanding of gender but need not detain us here. Instead we shall focus more on those people who require more significant assistance for ASC.

Similarly, many people have mild ID which does not require significant input and need not affect their gender, except perhaps to require more reasonably worded documents, explanations, and so forth (never a bad result to strive for in any case). Again, we shall not trouble unduly with this group here, but instead after we have considered ASC, we shall focus on those people for whom ID is a significant factor, especially in the case of capacity and consent.

Childhood Presentations

Parents and other caregivers of trans folk with ASC often report that there was 'no sign' of gender dysphoria earlier in childhood. It is said that no cross-sex behaviour, no cross-dressing, nothing unduly feminine or masculine ever presented itself before. It is often feared that the expressed gender dysphoria represents another of the many sorts of 'special interests' that came and went, intensely pursued and believed to be timeless and vital before waning and being discarded. Caregivers think that this too will diminish with time and that drastic and irreversible interventions will later be much regretted. These concerns are entirely understandable but are often misplaced.[1]

While we don't wish to stray too far into considering children here, it is worth noting that if caregivers are not accepting of gender diversity, young people learn that expressing their gender will be met with opprobrium. Thus the lack of cross-gender expression in the young person may be due to the caregivers, rather than the young person themself. Ironically when a caregiver expresses their opposition extremely vociferously and intrusively because no history was evident to them, it can actually lend weight to the young person's assertion that they did not feel safe to express themselves and that this is the real reason for their lack of apparent history.

Further, gender dysphoric teenagers with ASC very often don't express their gender, especially if it is atypical. Rather, they are often unusual in that they present in an unsexualised way: they are the only girl who hasn't tried to roll up her school uniform skirt to make it shorter, as the rules forbid and everyone does, and who doesn't see how much make-up they can get away with. They are the only boy who hasn't tried to contort the school uniform, by some means or another, into something at least slightly less drab. They wear the uniform as a *uniform*, plain and simple. They follow the rules[2] (and are the only ones not to try to bend those rules). This serves to delight the school, relieve their parents, and render them an irredeemable nerd in the eyes of their peers, which may or may not bother them very much.

Outside school, in a civilian setting so to speak, something similar happens in that there is often a slightly drab, gender-neutral clothing choice; sometimes a very stereotypical male or female choice (copied from others and worn entirely without panache or enjoyment); and occasionally bizarre but not particularly gendered choices based on preferences for

---

[1] Unfortunately, when caregivers read statements of this sort they almost inevitably think that it is their charge who is the exception rather than a member of the majority. Statistically, of course, this cannot be so, but sadly feeling is seldom a respecter of logic. It can nonetheless be worth explaining this and investigating in what way – other than the caregiver's strong conviction – their charge could be exceptional.

[2] Unless the rules are irredeemably unreasonable.

particular textures, colours, or whatever on the basis of the sensory hypersensitivities often seen in ASC.

Being the caregivers of children with ASC can be very difficult. There are so very many worries for the future and an acute awareness of so many vulnerabilities that the children themselves are wholly blind to. Things get even more worrying, of course, when children with gender dysphoria and ASC become aware – often through the internet – that they are not, in fact, entirely obliged to follow rigid rules on gender presentation defined by their sex assigned at birth. This necessarily sudden awareness of no such obligation tends to be rapidly followed by different gender expression. Sometimes this happens online at first (a realm caregivers are usually excluded from) and later in offline peer groups before bursting into domestic life, seemingly fully formed and all the more alarming as a consequence. It can usually be distinguished from an intense or special interest or obsession (of which there may have been several previously) because a special interest is in a subject, thing, or activity which is usually external to the self, whilst this is something to do with expressing oneself, located within individual identity and not external to it.

It should be noted that younger trans people with ASC (and indeed sometimes those who are neurotypical) sometimes initially declare that they are gay or lesbian, only later for this to mutate into a trans or non-binary presentation, perhaps as a testing of the parental waters, so to speak, or as a means of graded exposure to their own anxiety.

Diagnosis

Trans people with ASC present challenges not so much in diagnosis as in what follows from diagnosis. These include the practicalities of accomplishing a change in social gender role, coping with the inevitable lack of predictability in the extent of any welcome changes that might be expected from endocrine treatment, negotiating social and intimate relationships in a different gender role, and securing independence including in a work setting.

Sexuality

Sexuality in general is discussed in Chapter 8, *Sexuality, Relationships, and Reproduction*, but we shall consider a few matters pertinent to ASC here, as sexuality in ASC is not often enough discussed, possibly because caregivers are too embarrassed and also have very many other aspects of their charge's daily lives to worry about. Emotional and physical development are often not synchronised as they would be in neurotypical people, leaving parents and carers with the difficulty of discussing sexual matters with a pubertal person who may have the emotional development of somebody very much younger. This is a daunting prospect and the task often seems to be ducked, quite understandably if not wisely.

Some people with ASC do not form close, intimate relationships and their sexual life, if any, is likely to be expressed exclusively through private masturbation. Trans folk with ASC are frequently decidedly ill at ease with their own body and consequently are even less likely to form intimate relationships. Many find masturbating difficult and disturbing, often lacking the capacity to imagine themselves as having another sort of body whilst masturbating and consequently not bothering at all.

Treatment, particularly a change of social gender role and hormone treatment, decidedly alters this for many trans folk with ASC. Trans men treated with androgens often experience a hugely increased libido and trans women may also experience an increase in libido as their comfort with their body increases. An increased sense of authenticity in their social gender role and an increasing satisfaction with their own body lead many trans folk with ASC to make their first forays into sexual behaviour, including sexual behaviour with others, after such treatment has commenced. This can be a source of alarm for parents and carers who have previously viewed them, perhaps with some relief, as not particularly sexual beings.

Newly emerging sexual behaviour in trans folk with ASC can cause difficulties of three rather distinct sorts. The first is that the behaviour is sometimes the sort of experimental, adolescent venture usually seen in people very much younger and can be viewed as eccentric or even threatening when displayed by somebody much older than those normally expressing it.

A separate problem is that people with ASC may not be particularly circumspect about their trans status – certainly less cautious than those without ASC. Attempting to elicit sexual liaisons with an explicit mention of trans status from the outset tends to draw responses from [almost exclusively] men with a particular sexual interest in trans women. It is unlikely that lasting, mutually supportive relationships will come from such origins. Even if such relationships do persist, they have a tendency to abruptly dissolve once the patient has undergone genital surgery. Notably, people with ASC often prefer to contract relationships online at first and dating websites seem something of a happy hunting ground for men who seek trans women for sexual liaisons.

The third potential concern is that people with ASC, whether or not trans, seem more likely to enjoy consensual sadomasochistic sex and relationships (cf. Chapter 8, *Sexuality, Relationships, and Reproduction*; Richards & Barker, 2013). On closer inspection, this is entirely understandable. Among the major difficulties with more conventional relationships are the social uncertainties and finely balanced niceties that have to be gone through before things progress to the stage of any sexual interaction. This delicate *pas de deux* is even more difficult for those with ASC and is sometimes impossibly so. A sadomasochistic sexual life, on the other hand, is very much more straightforward in that there are, most definitely, *rules* (see Richards & Barker, 2013). If one wants sex, one goes to particular places, wears particular clothing, and can determine in advance of any intimate interaction exactly what will and will not occur and how one might control that, both beforehand and as the encounter progresses.

For parents and carers who have previously viewed their child or charge as a reassuringly rule-following, somehow sexless being, it can be difficult to cope, in quick succession, with a declaration of intention to change gender role, the change of such role, the onset of hormone treatment, and then a newly discovered desire to make intimate relationships. An emerging consensual sadomasochistic sexual lifestyle can be an alarming 'last straw' often directly attributed to a gender role change and hormone treatment when, in truth, the situation is more complex and the sadomasochism is more in keeping with the ASC – gender dysphoria having, in fact, prevented its earlier expression or, indeed, the expression of any particular sexuality at all.

People Severely Affected by ASC in Combination with Intellectual Disability – Institutional Responses

Institutional responses to apparent, emerging, or disclosed gender dysphoria have the potential to greatly help or equally hinder trans folk who are more disabled by their ASC and who consequently live in an institutional setting. Traditionally, and to a distressing extent currently, disabled people generally, and learning disabled people particularly, have tended to be viewed as essentially childlike beings with no sexual aspects to their character and no sexual expression in their lives. In a small proportion of cases, this perception is somewhat reasonable, particularly in those with endocrine abnormalities. Most of the time, however, it is not, and the desire for sexual expression or at the very least considerable intimacy is very much present and should be facilitated.

More recently, there has been more widespread acknowledgement of sexual desires and drives in people with learning disability and ASC – the general principle seems to have been that whilst such desires or activities are perfectly all right in themselves, they are 'private' and to be done in 'private' places. Although an increase in tolerance might be thought widespread, it is striking how often this seemingly more enlightened attitude is sorely tested, sometimes to the point of destruction, if it emerges that same-sex relations are what is wanted or if even mildly unusual, although perfectly legal, sexual desires are expressed.

Trans folk who also have ASC and learning disabilities and attempt to express themselves in this way in an institutional setting often have such expression viewed by their caregivers as primarily sexual in origin. Sometimes people with an intellectual disability speak about it using these terms themselves, not having heard any alternative formulation in the discourse of those around them and consequently lacking the vocabulary or articulation to provide any more accurate description of their motivation. They are often told that such behaviour as cross-dressing is "private behaviour" (the same as sexual behaviour) and that whilst it is not wrong, it is definitely should be done "in your private room" and not elsewhere.

For people required to keep such non-sexual behaviour 'private', after an initial, 'honeymoon' period, disruption and distress sadly often follow. The person concerned is often pleased at first to be able to express themselves in a more authentic way but to an almost equal and opposite degree grows increasingly to hate being required to return to their former gender role, particularly in a public way. It is definitely a case of half a loaf being most decidedly not better than none but rather a recurrent and upsetting reminder that a whole loaf of bread is being withheld.

Staff in institutions frequently express resistance when anyone with ASC presses for a more public presentation in their preferred gender role. It is often suggested that to do so would disturb or confuse other residents; there is also possibly a fear that sexuality might be more generally aroused in such a community. Increasingly disturbed behaviour often results, as the person with ASC presses their point until, eventually, and sometimes after several years, a half-hearted referral to a gender identity clinic is made.

Referrals such as these are often almost apologetically made, and it is sometimes clear that the accompanying staff anticipate the role of the clinic as one in which the person with ASC has it more carefully explained to them, by an authority figure, that this disturbed behaviour must cease, at least in public. Of course in some cases, it may be that the person is not, in fact, trans but another diagnosis pertains (see Chapter 2, *Assessment*). In many cases there is often some bemusement when a careful assessment is made, not uncommonly over multiple interviews; this may be followed by incredulity when it is suggested that the behaviour is not indicative of disturbed sexuality but rather a genuine feeling of gender dysphoria. The greatest difficulty comes when it is suggested that a formal change of gender role be actively considered. For a specialist consultant psychiatrist or consultant psychologist, it often feels that the hardest work is with the caregivers rather than the person with ASC. Getting care staff to genuinely and wholeheartedly embrace and facilitate a change of social gender role for someone with ASC is difficult; if it can be achieved, a very considerable improvement in behaviour and simultaneous improvement in the happiness and general functional abilities of the person with ASC is likely to take place. (As with people with mental illnesses and people who offend, endeavouring to assist while stressing the person through suppressing their genuine gender seldom works – see Chapter 5, *Supporting Trans and Non-binary People in Mental Health Services*, and Chapter 6, *Forensic Settings*, respectively). These improvements are often fairly quickly manifested, and once they become apparent, the increased cooperation of staff often follows. A second phase of difficulty, however, often occurs when the person with ASC wishes to present in their new social gender role in settings outside the relatively sequestered environment of that institution. A renegotiation of rather similar hurdles to those which had to be surmounted earlier sometimes reoccurs.

Some people in these circumstances will need advice and assistance with personal presentation. If this is the case, it is important that advisors do not make the mistake of advising 'dressing down for personal protection'. Very often people with pronounced ASC have for many years been socially marginalised figures, and the degree of social margin-alisation does not seem to increase with a change of social gender role but rather to decrease because personal confidence is greater and the ability to socially interact proportionally improved. Indeed, humans appear to have evolved to notice anxiety in others – probably as a means of spotting potential threat to themselves. Consequently, a misguided attempt to reduce threat by explaining danger and the need to 'dress down' to the person with ASC can lead to their being more anxious and uncomfortable, and so more noticeable and more under threat than if they had simply worn the [gendered] clothing they wished to.

Making New Friends as a Trans Person with ASC

At any one time, most of us have circles of people around us who provide comfort; to whom we are not biologically related; and with whom we fairly frequently associate for reasons that are not to do with commercial transaction (we don't buy things from them or sell things to them), not service related (they are not paid by us or someone else to do things to us or for us); and are not work related in that we don't currently work with them or, if we do, we see them outside of work as well as in a work setting. These people would be happy to lend small sums of money to us in the event of an emergency, and we would be prepared to lend to them in such circumstances. They would be happy for us to come into their homes and extend such invitations to us. Correspondingly, we would be happy for them to come into our homes.

The people described here are a supportive circle of friends, and such circles are one of the factors that sustain most people through their lives. Friendships are often formed in work or leisure settings where people meet – and they may persist even when the original reason for contact has long gone. Friends made at school may be lifelong; friendships made at work may persist when both people left that particular employer many years before.

There is a gradual 'churn' of friendships over the course of anyone's lifetime, some gradually ebbing away and others forming as life's various stages are passed. Friendships often end with geographical moves and changes of circumstances on the part of either party. Neurotypical people acquire new friends at around the same rate as old ones are lost, maintaining a broadly similar number at any one time over the course of many years. The number of friends anyone has tends to be particular to that person – some having many and others rather fewer closer, friends.

People with ASC often find it much harder to accrue friends than do neurotypical people, but their friendships are just as likely to be lost through changes in location or personal circumstances. Over time, even if there is a reasonable friendship group in the first place (often formed at school or work), the friendship circle becomes progressively smaller, and, as a consequence, the opportunities to acquire new friends proportionally diminish. Unfortunately, a change of social gender role on the part of a trans person with ASC is exactly the sort of change in circumstance likely to sever at least a proportion of their friendships. There may also be an associated geographical move and sometimes also a change in occupation or a period of unemployment – although these events are by no means necessary. They do, however, act to deplete the circle of friends.

Neurotypical people who have lost a social circle through a change of social gender role (or for any other reason, for that matter) tend to garner new friends without much conscious thought about how they do so. Indeed, forming new friendships by neurotypical people can be likened, in some ways, to a motor car with a stalled engine resting, motionless, at the top of a long, very shallow gradient. With a small amount of effort, such a car can be moved from a resting state to a gentle roll forward down the shallow slope. The car doesn't roll ever faster and faster because of rolling resistance and fairly quickly establishes a sedate, steady speed and rolls on indefinitely with no further efforts required.

A person with ASC, on the other hand, can be likened to an identical car but with under-inflated tyres that don't roll so easily because the rolling resistance is higher. Equally motionless at the outset, a considerably greater degree of effort is required to achieve any friend-gathering motion in the first place; if that motion is to be sustained, a perpetually continued, although mild, force must be applied to prevent the motion slowly petering out and stasis once again establishing itself.

In practical application, people with ASC who have changed their social gender role (or lost much of their social circle for any other reason, for that matter) have to make particular and conscious efforts to acquire new friends and will need to apply continued efforts thereafter, albeit at a much lower level, if they are not gradually to lose their friends through 'churn' faster than they can acquire them. It can therefore be worthwhile to consider what sorts of social venues would likely offer a fairly warm, non-judgmental, and tolerant welcome to somebody with ASC who has a changed social gender role. Four examples spring to mind and a little thought might produce several others.The first are religious groups, particularly those which are well established and have a reputation for tolerance and lack extreme dogmatism or a tendency to evangelise. The Religious Society of Friends (Quakers) or very mainstream branches of the Church of England leap to mind, as does the Metropolitan Church. Attendance at any such group carries with it many associated social activities; if the trans person is willing to assist in any way, a warm welcome is particularly likely. There are always premises to keep spick and span, tea to pour, elderly communicants to visit at home, flowers to arrange, grounds to maintain, and groups to convene. Quizzes must be organised; barn dances arranged. The traditional children's theatrical activity with three wise men and vast numbers of sheep and shepherds needs to be put on once a year. The diligence and tolerance of tedium sometimes found in those with ASC act as an asset on these occasions in that the welcome to the trans person is even warmer because of the secret hatred on the part of most everybody else for these particular tasks.

The second are political parties. The aim of all political parties is to acquire power and thus effect the changes they believe are imperative. This cannot be achieved without mass support and membership; consequently, virtually all political parties welcome members of any sort. Further, political parties can't retain members without offering about 60% social and 40% political activities. Membership of almost any political party seems inevitably to involve hours spent chatting while stuffing campaign literature into envelopes; further hours spent in a bar discussing the merits of this, that, or another initiative or person within the party; and companionable evenings stumping around rain-sodden streets, knocking on doors to promote the Great Cause before a foot-weary collapse into the pub for what might very loosely be termed "a debrief". The sense of a common cause, shared tasks, external enemies, and adversities are exactly what promotes feelings of unity and friendship. Such friendships tend to follow whatever political party is joined, although it does seem sensible to pick one with at least a reasonable accord with one's personal views.

A third is the local amateur dramatic society. The desire to tread the theatrical boards seems so widespread a drive that few places in the United Kingdom, and indeed many places in other countries, are not within easy reach of an amateur dramatic society. The kinds of people such societies attract are often unlikely to be bothered by sexual or gender differences. Instead, such groups throng with outgoing, gregarious individuals whose every moment outside work seems to revolve around the stage. Evenings spent in a theatre bar may leave the trans person feeling surrounded by a multitude of skilled monologues, each delighted to have found a new audience of one. Welcome above all is someone willing to paint sets, construct scenery, repair and create costumes, source props, serve drinks, herd bovine audiences, rig or operate sound and lighting equipment, act as prompt, or be assistant stage manager (that most Herculean of tasks). In time, even the shyest of trans people might be cajoled into appearing in Act 2 to say "the doctor has arrived, Mr Blenkinsop."

Last, but by no means least, there are, of course, LGBT or trans-specific support groups, both online and offline. These can be absolutely invaluable, as they offer actual understanding and targeted specific support. The only slight caveat is that some people with a predisposition to feel threatened can use them as a sort of 'safety behaviour', assuming that only LGBT people will be accepting and that heterosexual cisgender people will not. People can limit themselves to LGBT spaces when, in fact, they would be quite welcome in the sorts of places everyone goes to such as those listed earlier. Because people who feel under threat do not test out whether or not they would be welcome in mainstream life, they can be unnecessarily limited. LGBT groups can be amazing places to shelter from the storm, but when the sun is out, so to speak, it is not usually the best outcome for them to be the *only* place one resides. Of course, the best result is to have the option to go to both LGBT- and non-LGBT-specific places and attend whichever one wishes at the time.

Getting Help with Appearance

Because trans people with ASC have an impaired theory of mind, they are less likely to have an acute awareness of how others see them and what thoughts and feelings their appearance provokes. Some trans people with ASC can become rather frustrated because they are fully aware of their own gender and have made little effort to communicate that gender to others through appearance. Consequently, others remain *un*aware of the trans person's gender, with the confusion and frustration this naturally bring to the trans person.

For a trans person with ASC, appearance in their birth-assigned gender role is very often the product of previous longer-term parental or sibling advice that might not be available after a change of social gender role in adult life, particularly if family relations have broken down or there has been an abandonment by the initial social group. In such instances, it's worthwhile for trans people to look at what other people of their gender role, age, general build, and appearance are wearing and taking advice from friends or professional shop assistants.

It can be helpful in some cases to gently but firmly point out that if one is a cisgender woman who looks petite and elfin (like the young Audrey Hepburn or Sinead O'Connor,[3] for example), then wearing a donkey jacket and heavy work boots serves only, in some peculiar way, to emphasise one's waif-like femininity. If, on the other hand, one has a more substantial build, then wearing those clothes is unlikely to make one look more feminine but rather like someone who has come to supervise some road diggers. With a substantial build comes a need for clothing styles which flatter a larger size, while giving sufficient cues as to one's gender for the response one seeks. It is worthwhile considering too that many cisgender women are of a more substantial build, rather than being a young Audrey Hepburn or Sinead O'Connor.

A number of major clothing stores offer a service whereby staff will select clothes for an individual, according to budget or for a specific event. For trans women, particularly, the issue is not so much a single event but more the acquisition of appropriate clothes for the wide variety of events she is likely to encounter in the immediate to medium future, and this too can be accommodated. The service is usually entirely without charge and can be booked online from the store's website, which will automatically direct the shopper to the nearest store that offers this service.

Similar advice follows with hairdressers and barbers. By and large, they are interested and helpful if they are told exactly what your situation is (and if they are not, trans and non-binary folk can give their custom to plenty of others). Trans-feminine people who have some head hair loss should be advised that countless thousands of cisgender women have exactly the same problem; as a result, hairdressers are often expert at coming up with ingenious solutions, provided they have an honestly presented story of what is needed.

In a related vein, excellent and free advice is available from those people employed at the make-up counter in most big department stores. Seemingly always dressed in sparking white tunics, for some reason, their job is to persuade passing customers to buy make-up. Their job is to show customers what wonders can be created with the products in the expectation that they will buy the products to recreate the effect at home. They are really well trained, of course, and if a trans-feminine person approaches them and ask to have her make-up done, they will almost always ask what occasion the make-up is for. Is it for a glamorous evening in a poorly lit bar or a daytime, daylight job interview? Is it the kind of bulletproof make-up that has to stand a long-haul plane flight to a tropical country or are the circumstances such that touch-ups are possible? The answer, of course, is all of these and more. If the circumstances are explained to them, they will usually exert their skills, in part because theirs can sometimes be a boring job and the trans-feminine person represents an interesting change to the ordinary run of things. It's a good idea when they have finished for the customer to use her phone to photograph the results from the front, sides, and quarter view because a mirror only shows us from the front, whilst

---

[3] Younger readers please sigh and insert your own example as you see fit.

others see us from the side, as well. When they have finished doing the make-up in five ways for five sorts of occasion, the trans-feminine person can, if she wishes, buy the make-up to use herself at home.

Discrimination

Trans people are at a greater risk of discrimination than cisgender people. This should not be overstated, as discrimination is by no means inevitable (see Chapter 1, *Introduction*), but it does occur. Naturally, intersections of marginalisation matter here. If one is white, wealthy, able-bodied, and so on, one usually has far fewer difficulties with discrimination than if one is none of those things. It follows, therefore, that trans people with ASC and/or ID will experience greater discrimination than those without – this can be particularly the case if the nature of the condition means that the trans person is less able to avoid, or respond to, abuse. Psychiatrists and psychologists can usefully provide, or refer for, skills in managing conflict and can also use their professional power to underscore that gender diversity is absolutely OK – a useful message if the person has been told by another person with some degree of authority that it is not. It should almost go without saying that any staff in a clinical setting who are not accepting of gender diversity in principle will benefit from robust assistance towards change from psychiatrists, psychologists, and others such as human resource personnel. Such discrimination can never be justified by personal belief of course; when one is at work one is expected to fulfil that role – one's personal beliefs are just that – a personal rather than a professional matter.

Summary

Trans people with ASC and/or ID have specific needs both related and unrelated to their gender status. These needs, associated as they are with both cognition and social interaction, can constrain people from being able to fully express themselves, and from being able to easily navigate the sometimes difficult social world which arises when they do. Naturally, not expressing oneself is not an option which leads to an unproblematic outcome – leading, as it sadly almost inevitably does, to increased distress and decompensation. Certainly any endeavours towards pro-social behaviours and development will almost certainly be doomed to failure if the person one is working with is unable to express such a fundamental part of themselves.

The general clinical environment should naturally be adapted to be accommodating of people with ASC and/or ID and should also be accommodating of trans people (see Chapter 1, *Introduction*); therefore, it should also be accommodating of the relatively high numbers of people who have ASC and/or ID and who are also trans. Psychiatrists and psychologists are encouraged to also give thought as to how they may equip their patients to manage the vicissitudes of life outside of the clinic, and further to directly advocate for policy changes and laws to improve that environment more generally.

Further Reading

Glidden, D., Bouman, W. P., Jones, B. A., & Arcelus, J. (2016). Gender dysphoria and autism spectrum disorder: A systematic review of the literature. *Sexual Medicine Reviews*, 4(1), 3–14.

Richards, C. (2015). Further sexualities. In C. Richards & M. J. Barker (eds.). *The*

Palgrave handbook of the psychology of sexuality and gender (pp. 60–76). London: Palgrave-Macmillan.

Richards, C., & Barker. M. (eds.) (2013). *Sexuality and gender for mental health professionals: A practical guide*. London: Sage.

References

Richards, C., & Barker. M. (eds.) (2013). *Sexuality and gender for mental health professionals: A practical guide*. London: Sage.

Sexuality, Relationships, and Reproduction

8

Introduction

It is sometimes supposed that sexuality and gender are directly causal or at least fundamentally intertwined – that is, that a person who is female must be sexually attracted to men and conversely that those who are male must be attracted to women. Thus if a person is a trans woman, it is supposed she will be attracted to men; accordingly, trans men will be attracted to women. While this is true in many cases, it is by no means invariably so, as, of course, many men are attracted to men, and many women are attracted to women – gay men and lesbian women, respectively, as well as bisexual or pansexual people. This remains the case for trans people who have slightly higher rates of non-heterosexual attraction as a group, most likely because trans people have necessarily considered their gender, which naturally leads to wider consideration of other matters including sexuality (and also relationships, employment, reproduction, and so on).

Of course trans people may have a non-binary gender rather than a binary one and – irrespective of gender – trans people may be bisexual or pansexual – that is, they may be attracted to people irrespective of gender. Trans people, as with cisgender people, may also have a wide variety of other sexualities such as engaging in the consensual exchange of power or sensation (BDSM – bondage and discipline, dominance and submission, and sadomasochism), fetishism, and so on (see Richards, 2015).

As we have noted, sexuality is generally decoupled from gender; however, in some instances is it *lexically* coupled – for example, to be a lesbian one must be attracted to women and also be a woman. Such is not the case where a person is bisexual, of course. However, in instances where the gender of the person someone is attracted to is known, but their own gender is not, there are two useful terms – *gynephile* (attracted to women) and *androphile* (attracted to men), although this is not necessarily helpful for those people attracted to non-binary people.

We will not unduly consider heterosexuality, bisexuality, or solely same-sex attraction separately here, as we would hope the reader is adequately versed in these sexualities and so is able to apply the principles to trans people. We should note, however, the difference between *identity* and *practice*: some people – both trans and cisgender – have identities which differ from their practices and some engage in practices which differ from their identities. This is because identities have aspects to them aside from the pure elements of any associated practice. For example, many people drive a car (Practice) but are not Petrolheads (Identity), as they do not read magazines about the latest cars, follow the latest car releases, and so on. Similarly, many people play games on their phone (Practice) but are not Gamers (Identity); indeed, some gamers may not actually be playing games due to work or family commitments but may still identify as Gamers and follow the latest tech and gaming news. In terms of sexuality, many men have sex with men (Practice) but may not be Gay (Identity); many people identify as Gay or as Heterosexual (Identity) but may not be in a relationship or having sexual intercourse (Practice). In sum, it is important not to confuse what people are *doing* with who they *are* (and vice versa). We will discuss some trans specific matters pertaining to this later, but for more information, see Richards and Barker (2013) and Richards et al. (2019). Instead, here we will touch upon some misunderstood sexualities and how they interact with trans – namely, BDSM and fetishism – before moving on to other forms of relationships and reproduction.

BDSM – Bondage and Discipline, Dominance and Submission, and Sadomasochism

BDSM, or *kink* as it is also colloquially known, consists of the consensual exchange of power and/or sensation. Note the inclusion of *consensual* here, as the principle is central. Most practitioners practise Risk Aware Consensual Kink (the delightfully named RACK) in which the management of risk and the focus on consensuality are the key components. If it is not consensual it is not BDSM; it is rape – just as non-consensual Heterosexual Penis-in-Vagina (PiV)[1] sex stops being sleeping together (or another term) and becomes rape.

It is worth considering that compared to BDSM spanking say, PiV sex is highly risky – being the transmission route for most STIs and the only form of sexual contact with a high risk of unwanted pregnancy. Given the relative risk compared to PiV sex, and that there is no necessary dysfunction, BDSM is no longer considered pathological. The DSM retains the diagnoses 'sexual masochism disorder' and 'sexual sadism disorder' but only if there are "Clinically significant distress to the individual or impairment in social, occupational, or other important areas of functioning" (p. 694) – simply having BDSM as a sexual interest is insufficient to merit a diagnosis. The ICD 11 has taken this a step further and has removed sexual masochism entirely, and only includes sexual sadism if it is *coercive* (as *6D33 Coercive Sexual Sadism Disorder*) so is quite different from the matters under discussion here. One might consider *6D36 Paraphilic Disorder involving Solitary Behaviour or Consenting Individuals*, which very sensibly does not identify specific behaviours considered suspect. However, one of the criteria is that "The person is markedly distressed by the nature of the arousal pattern and the distress is not simply a consequence of rejection or feared rejection of the arousal pattern by others" (WHO, 2019a), a statement made in the context of the fact that distress about BDSM in the absence of rejection by others is vanishingly rare.

We include this minor detour into BDSM here to underscore the evolving nature of such diagnoses, and because it is not uncommon for trans people, as with cisgender people, to engage with this (Holvoet et al., 2017). Trans people especially may use BDSM to explore gender roles within a safely defined space where boundaries and expectations are explicitly agreed beforehand.[2] Having made this first step, some trans people may then take the plunge into the wider world in a non-sexual way; indeed, in some instances BDSM itself is non-sexual but rather a forum for the exploration of sensation, identity, and power. We must therefore be careful not to assume a sexual basis for a gender which has had its first expression in a [sometimes] sexual space.

---

[1] Or vagina-surrounding-penis.
[2] In both senses of the word 'explicitly'.

Fetishism

There is a close cross-over between BDSM and fetishism in that many people in BDSM spaces may enjoy wearing rubber or leather or have other preferences for sexual acts or sensations. For our purposes here, we shall consider sexual excitement associated with wearing clothing not normally worn by people of that birth-assigned sex. Of course, this is a somewhat antediluvian understanding of clothing, and of fetishism, as so much clothing is now androgynous; nonetheless, *when associated with sexual excitement* wearing clothing not normally worn by people of that birth-assigned sex is still codified in the DSM as *Transvestic Fetishism*, again with the caveat that "The fantasies, sexual urges, or behaviours [must] cause clinically significant distress or impairment in social, occupational, or other important areas of functioning" (APA, 2013, p. 702). The question naturally arises as to why this potential cause of dysfunction is listed and not others such as 'financial insufficiency disorder' (if we are listing causes, rather than symptoms or syndromes; cf Richards, 2015). Especially as in this instance it is usually social opprobrium and not the act of wearing clothing itself which is psychopathogenic. The answer given by Spitzer (the convenor of the DSM IV-TR) is that removal would have been a "public relations disaster for psychiatry" (cited in Kleinplatz & Moser, 2005, p. 137). The World Health Organization nonetheless believed it could weather such a 'disaster', and so 'transvestism' of any sort is no longer included in the *International statistical classification of diseases and related health problems version 11* (WHO, 2019b).

Some trans people, perhaps especially those who are a little older and who have spent a good deal of time in a traditional gender role assigned at birth, may have a quite lengthy period where dressing in clothing usually worn by another gender is sexually arousing (usually people assigned male at birth wearing 'women's clothing'). This may then shift away from sexuality and towards a feeling of comfort, before finally shifting to a wish to *be* another gender. This group of people can go on to do quite well after surgery or hormones if they have spent time living in their identified gender role and if the sexual drive for transition is now quite absent. The risk arises where the sexual drive for transition remains.

The risk of a sexual drive for transition leading to actual transition is due to the fact that the sexual excitement comes from the juxtaposition of the male and the female – it is being a *man* wearing women's clothes which is exciting. The person may think it will be even more exciting to actually *be* and live as a woman and so is motivated to seek physical changes (often abroad) and spend their life as a woman. However, they are then effectively a woman living as a woman, which loses the erotic tension and, as time wears on and the excitement of being a woman attenuates, the person is left without the motivation for transition but having made permanent changes. For this reason, current sexual arousal associated with cross-dressing is a contraindication to hormones or surgeries. This is caveated with the fact that the sexuality may shift as detailed earlier and may be the first part of an exploration as detailed in the section on BDSM.

As the sexual arena is the first space for exploration of gender for some trans people, a small number who are used to expressing their gender in clubs and parties can misunderstand the nature of the clinical encounter with a psychiatrist or psychologist – feeling that it is an extension of the option for the very expressive behaviours they have exhibited elsewhere. It may be necessary to gently explain that this is a professional encounter, just as when they discuss an orthopaedic matter or something similar, even to express the limits on acceptable dress in your clinic. Don't be overly concerned, however, as in general trans people will wear entirely appropriate attire, although just sometimes if still in a process of transition, a little younger than one might expect as people try out different styles to see which suits.

Relationships

Trans people have all the different relationship structures one might expect, including marriage, civil partnerships, informal relationships, and monogamy (see Chapter 9, *Legal and Religious Aspects*, for details of the legal hurdles). The most common relationship structures are those one might expect to see for cisgender people – and any assumption that a trans person will necessarily not be able to find a stable happy relationship by reason of being trans is false, as are assumptions that relationships must invariably fail if a person transitions. Certainly, there can be a significant period of adjustment for some, but for younger people – increasing numbers of whom identify as queer rather than heterosexual – there appears to be far less (or no) adjustment than for people who have grown up in other time periods.

In general, problems can arise when one partner is heterosexual and is simply not sexually attracted to the person who has transitioned. In the United Kingdom, this tends to be fairly amicably resolved, with a strong friendship remaining after the partners have separated and sought another person they are sexually attracted to. Again, separation is not invariably the case, especially when there is no homophobia and sex is not central to the relationship prior to the transition.

Problems do arise, however, in couples where being 'Normal'[3] is vital to their self-worth and who have a brittle sense of self and relationship. Here the work is usually not about being trans (although transphobia will need to be addressed), but about being comfortable with being outside the exact centre of whatever the couple imagine the social or cultural mainstream to be. Very often the couple have expended very significant emotional and financial effort to appear 'Normal' and the fear both of what lies outside that tight delineation and also that all that effort might have been unnecessary (cf Richards, 2010), can be intolerable. Significant psychotherapy can be of assistance here; however, very often the non-transitioning partner situates the problem solely in the trans partner, which means that the *couple* are not amenable to therapy, although it is the couple which are key.

Further, the trans person themselves may feel guilty for having 'hurt' their partner by being trans. This is misplaced, as there was usually no deceit involved and the trans person did not intend to be trans – indeed, there is nothing wrong with being trans at all. Nonetheless, the trans person points to the 'hurt' and suggests that they should feel guilt for hurting their partner (or children, parents, etc.). However, the partner need *not* be hurt – it is not inevitable that they will be so, as we have seen, many partners are not. This implies that it is the trans person (the nature of any transition), their partner (their response to their partner being trans), and also the relationship which needs addressing.

We might consider the analogy of a woman, Sue, shooting a man, Peter, in the leg – in this instance, Sue is hurting Peter – there is no other reasonable response to being shot in the leg than being hurt. But, alternatively, let us consider a woman, Jane, working as a newsagent, and a man, Gerald, outraged that a woman is working when she should be at home. Here Jane has 'hurt' Gerald but *his response might have been otherwise*. The situation of a partner transitioning is analogous to the second instance,

---

[3] Note the capital letter.

not the first (cf Richards & Barker, 2013). Making this clear (and indeed using this metaphor) can be the first step in moving forward. This is not to say that the partner should not feel what they do, but that it is not inevitably so – there is the possibility of change and healing and an exploration of the nature of the relationship going forward. The change may not lead to a perfect outcome. Sometimes all one can hope for is the 'least-worst' outcome as both partners adapt as best they can, but inevitably change there must be.

Aside from couple relationships, there are also trans people (and indeed cisgender people) who are in consensual relationships of more than two people. Again, consensuality is key here – this is not infidelity. These relationship structures are called polyamory or non-monogamies. Various 'rules' (all grounded in consent) are accepted – for some it is living together and sharing love, bills, housing, child-rearing, and so on (polyamory); for some, love is kept within the primary dyad, but sex is shared elsewhere – swinging, dogging, some other forms of non-monogamies (cf Easton & Liszt, 2017). Trans people may engage in any of these relationship structures. Having more than one other partner can be comfortable for some people with non-[gender] binary identities as there are more options for gender expression available with different people, but usually trans and cisgender people are polyamorous or non-monogamous because it feels right and suits emotional and sexual needs, just as monogamy does for others.

General Issues with Sexuality

Sexuality for trans people is not intrinsically bound up with gender or with the utility of body parts, but these things are tightly linked. For example, some trans people report sexuality changes through transition – often after a significant change such as social transition, starting cross-sex hormones, or after surgeries. For some, this can be a part of experimentation; for others, it comes as something of a surprise as new sexual interests emerge after a long period of settled sexuality. This can lead to a period of reflection and experimentation much as in the case of cisgender adolescents who are exploring sexuality; although as many trans people are already adults, it will naturally be leavened with the balanced approach available to people who have already matured.

One of the elements of exploration which may be undertaken is exploring desire and practice with new body parts and bodily sensations. This should be encouraged, as human sexuality is an important part of life for many people. It can take time to become comfortable and familiar with a new bodily habitus. It can also be useful to underline to people that there are many different way of having sex – speaking of sex only as PiV sex is to miss the many practices people undertake and may exclude those people who do not have those body parts, do not wish to have that form of sex, and may miss STI routes and safer sex discussions.

Psychiatrists and psychologists should also be aware that the meaning of body parts may be reinterpreted by trans people; for example, a trans man may not refer to his vagina (deeming that to be a woman's body part) but may refer to his *man hole*. Similarly, trans women may refer to their *clitoris*, rather than penis. At first blush, this may seem unusual; however, there is a long history of reinterpreting the meaning of masculine and feminine things – trousers for women are so usual as to no longer be of note in Western cultures; long hair is seen as feminine in some contexts but also as masculine in others (wrestlers, heavy metal musicians); male 'breast' cancer is seen in male chests, and so on. As ever, using the patient's own terminology is the best, and most polite, way to act. While there may be a need for medical specificity in some particular contexts, in general the patient's language can and should be respected, with a note appended if technically necessary.

One might (perhaps with an edge of sophistry) seek to extend the argument to suggest that surgeries are not needed as trans people can simply reinterpret their current body morphology. However, this does not work. As seen in Chapter 2, *Assessment*, talking to trans people with the firm intention of avoiding surgery (which is a quite different matter from assessing for surgery) does not work and is [therefore] unethical. Because one person is able to be comfortable with a reinterpreted body part does not mean another will – not least for the reason that if, for example, you wish to have receptive vaginal sex you need to have a vagina. Indeed, it is a common discourse from trans people that to access certain sexual spaces and relationships, a certain body is required. For instance, to feel comfortable in gay male bear spaces, people understandably feel the need to have male-typical body hair (see Richards, 2017).

Another form of 'sexuality' mentioned here (in much the same way that atheism is a form of 'religion') is asexuality. Asexual people usually do not experience sexual attraction. As always, there are variations beyond the strict definition, any of which have their own terminology. For example, there are people who are only sexual after significant romantic involvement; who are sexual in solo sex, but not with others; or who are sexual with partners due to the partner's preference and their own indifference rather than dislike. It is important not to immediately pathologise lack of sexual desire – a lack of desire may be part of another condition but is often dispositional. Good history taking as to how long they have been asexual and consideration of the patient's own views are vital. For our purposes here, there are also those people who are asexual until transition. There may be various reasons for this, but the simplest of them is that people do not experience desire for sex with another person if they are unable to express themselves sexually and will therefore be responded to inappropriately due to having a body morphology which does not reflect their identity.

Sex and Risk

While not all trans people wish to have sexual contact, many do wish to express themselves sexually, and for different reasons as we have seen. There are also a number of different contexts just as for cisgender people – as part of a loving relationship; as a form of recreation; as a commercial enterprise in the form of sex work; or as exploitation by others for personal, sexual, or financial gain. The latter of these is especially risky, and trans people may be especially at risk of being exploited due to being marginalised. Some trans people, especially those who are homeless, have mental health problems and/or substance misuse problems, may be coerced into sex work, or [usually falsely] believe that the sense of community sometimes found in sex work is the only source of support available to them. A multidisciplinary approach which addresses all of the issues in such cases is vital.

Some trans people may also engage in sex work as a means of obtaining enough money to pay for the hormones and surgeries which they are seeking. Fortunately, in countries such as the United Kingdom where healthcare is free at the point of delivery, this is far less of a necessity and trans people are therefore at less risk of exploitation through unwanted sex work – and therefore also STIs.

Sexually Transmitted Infections

STIs are, of course, still a risk for trans people for several reasons. One reason is that there may be an assumption that trans people on hormones or with surgically adapted body parts are unable to contract STIs. This is not the case; therefore, the Faculty of Sexual and Reproductive Healthcare of the Royal College of Obstetricians and Gynaecologists (FSRH) recommend that trans and non-binary individuals who engage in high-risk sexual behaviours should be sensitively advised about the importance of safer sex, including barrier methods and the availability of HIV PrEP (Pre-exposure Prophylaxis) and HIV PEPSE (Post-exposure Prophylaxis following sexual exposure) (FSRH, 2017). Some trans people may also be at greater risk of STIs due to the fact that they engage in risky sexual practices because they fear, or have been told, that their partner will leave them if they do not, and further that because they are trans they will therefore not be able to find another partner. This is decidedly not the case, as trans people very frequently have happy, healthy, fulfilling relationships – much though abusers may wish this were not the case.

Lastly, trans people may be reluctant to engage in STI testing due to the belief that it is unduly gendered. Indeed, this can still be the case; however, many STI clinics are now very accommodating of trans people and (correctly) consider body parts, sexual practices, and routes of transmission to be of primary importance, rather than the gender of the person they are engaging with and so order their clinics accordingly.

Fertility

Many of the treatments sought by trans and non-binary people affect or remove reproductive capacity. Cross-sex hormones are likely to remove reproductive capacity, but this is not guaranteed, consequently people should be counselled before starting hormones about gamete storage due to infertility *and* around using contraception. Because of the hormonal nature of much contraception (often using the very hormones the person is seeking to remove), barrier methods are usually the preferred method of contraception, although these too are by no means guaranteed to prevent STIs or pregnancy. The FSRH (2017) and British Association for Sexual Health and HIV (BASHH, 2019) have specific guidance on contraception for trans people. In general, combined hormonal methods are not suitable for trans men and non-binary people who take testosterone, but progestogen-only methods including emergency contraception, intrauterine system (IUS), or intrauterine device (IUD) may be used and should not interfere with their testosterone treatment.

Of course, if a person has a hysterectomy and oophorectomy (or orchidectomy), they will be rendered permanently infertile and such methods will prove unnecessary for contraception. Gamete storage in this case should be available just as it is for a cisgender person who has a diagnosed condition for whom the usual treatment removes reproductive capacity. Naturally certain sensitivities need to occur to make the trans person comfortable – a trans man would usually feel uncomfortable in a 'women's' fertility clinic. Happily, as with STI clinics, many fertility clinics are now making sensible arrangements to accommodate these patient groups, and appropriate wording in the referral may avert uncomfortable experiences.

There is sometimes the supposition that trans people do not want children or have somehow given up their right to have children through undergoing necessary medical treatments. These ideas are, of course, false. For a group of young trans people, however, matters become more complicated. Many young trans people seeking hormones are very much below the age at which people usually have children and often rather airily make the assertion at age 18 or so that they have "never wanted children" and therefore do not wish to store gametes before taking hormones. Of course, they are legally entitled to make such a decision, but may nonetheless come to regret it later in life. Some say they would adopt without being aware of what is involved – with some assuming one simply selects a neonate and gets on with it, which is very much not the case. Many younger trans people are focused only on the period of transition and wish to access hormones and surgeries as soon as possible, without considering the wider implications for their life post-transition – which will be vastly longer. It can be useful to make clear to them that ultimately they will only have to answer to themselves (it gets round the parental-type resistance), but that their older self will likely want them to have considered and researched the matter fully rather than allowing the thoughts of the 12- to 18-year-old who 'never wanted' children to dominate.

There are also those trans people who have taken hormones and have then stopped, whose fertility has [fortunately] returned. Thus there are increasing numbers of pregnant men, as well as women who have progenited their children with sperm. As ever, assumptions should not be made, and suitably accommodating services based upon need rather than gender are vital. Psychiatrists and psychologists may need to lead in instigating this sort of culture shift and service provision.

Children

Trans people may, of course, be children themselves, and this group is considered elsewhere. Here we consider the children of trans people, who do just as well as the children of their cisgender peers and indeed do not appear to be affected in terms of sexuality or gender either (White & Ettner, 2007). If a parent or caregiver is in the process of transition, this can often (although not always) create a period of significant change in the family. Where this is acrimonious (if a partner does not accept the transition, for example), there can be a negative effect upon children. However, this is not trans specific – acrimony between parents or caregivers for *any* reason has a negative effect. Some people opt to defer transition until children have grown up; however, this itself can create stress and secrecy in the family which can cause harm. Certainly asking children to hold secrets has been shown to be detrimental to them.

Some parents are concerned about their children being bullied at school, and indeed this can occur; however, it should not deter transition. Sadly some well-meaning social workers and others have not thought this through thoroughly and suggest they are acting "in the best interests of the child" to prevent a transition to retain access. Instead, the school should put into place robust anti-bullying measures just as they would if a child were being bullied for any other matter. To suggest that an adult, or group of adults, should not act because of the thoughts of a 7-year-old playground bully should be given the short shrift it so clearly deserves.

That said, some trans people do put off transition until children have reached a certain milestone and this can be sensible – telling children in the middle of exams may be unwise, for example. However, this can also be a means of deferring transition while keeping a comfortable idea that it will happen 'in the future'. The milestones often shift so "after starting school" becomes "after settled in", becomes "after secondary school", … GCSEs, … A-Levels, … university, … grandchildren born, … started school …. An honest conversation acknowledging these sensible concerns but also exploring fears can pay dividends.

Sometimes this deferral can be due to guilt, and sometimes for other reasons. Guilt experienced by transitioning parents or caregivers can be especially pernicious as they can feel that they have 'hurt' their children (see earlier discussion) but also that they must not stop feeling guilty as then they *would no longer feel guilty for having 'hurt' their children* – which would make them an even worse parent. In other words, to be a good parent, they must continue to feel guilty. Psychiatrists and psychologists can assist these groups of people by reassuring them that they are not guilty for being trans (as it is likely innate) and indeed that there is nothing to be 'guilty' *for* – the distress of their child is not their fault any more than if they had a physical health condition.

Summary

As psychiatrists and psychologists, we often feel more comfortable speaking about mental illness than mental and physical wellness, and too often we avoid sexuality entirely. This is unfortunate, as these conversations reveal more of our patients' lives which allow us to assist with wellness, identify strengths, and avoid mistakes which might potentially sabotage patient rapport. Talking gently and candidly about sexuality, using ordinary terms and an ordinary tone of voice can be invaluable for all patients, and perhaps in particular for trans people. Undue attention should not be paid to trans people's genitals and sexuality (or indeed anyone's genitals and sexuality); trans people are very much more than the contents of their underwear and become very tired of intrusive questions such as "have you had the operation yet?" Unless it is absolutely pertinent to one's work, such questions should not be asked. This is quite different, of course, from asking if a person has a partner or partners – a quite usual question which will build rapport. Trans people may have partners who are cisgender, transgender, non-binary; may be sexual or asexual; and may have a variety of practices and identities. As psychiatrists and psychologists, we can be respectful of these things and so provide more effective care.

Further Reading

Richards, C., & Barker. M. (2013). *Sexuality and gender for mental health professionals: A practical guide*. London: Sage.

(2014). Trans and existentialism. In M. Milton (ed.). *Sexuality: Existential perspectives* (pp. 217–230). Ross-on-Wye: PCCS Books.

Richards, C., & Barker, M. J. (eds.). (2015). *The Palgrave handbook of the psychology of sexuality and gender*. London: Palgrave-Macmillan.

Richards, C., Bouman, W. P., & Barker, M. J. (eds.). (2018). *Genderqueer and non-binary genders*. London: Palgrave-Macmillan.

Richards, C., Farndon, H., Gibson, S., Jamieson, R., Moon, I., Lenihan, P., Rimes, K., & Semlyen, J. (2019). *Guidelines for psychologists working with gender, sexuality and relationship diversity* (2nd ed.). London: British Psychological Society.

References

American Psychiatric Association (APA). (2013). *Diagnostic and statistical manual of mental disorders 5*. Washington DC: American Psychiatric Association.

British Association for Sexual Health and HIV (BASHH). (2019). *Recommendations for integrated sexual health services for trans, including non-binary, people*. Cheshire: BASHH.

Easton, D., & Liszt, C. A. (2017). *The ethical slut* (3rd ed.). San Francisco: Greenery Press.

The Faculty of Sexual and Reproductive Health Care of the Royal College of Obstetricians and Gynaecologists (FSRH) (2017). *Contraceptive choices and sexual health for transgender non-binary people*. London: FSRH.

Holvoet, L., Huys, W., Coppens, V., Seeuws, J., Goethals, K., & Morrens, M. (2017). Fifty shades of Belgian gray: The prevalence of BDSM-related fantasies and activities in the general population. *The Journal of Sexual Medicine, 14* (9), 1152–1159.

Kleinplatz, P. J., & Moser, C. (2005). Politics versus science: An addendum and response to Drs Spitzer and Fink. In D. Karasic & J. Drescher (eds.), *Sexual and gender diagnoses of the diagnostic and statistical manual (DSM)* (pp. 91–109). New York: The Haworth Press.

Richards, C. (2010). 'Them and us' in mental health services. *The Psychologist, 23* (1). 40–41.

(2015). Further sexualities. In Richards, C., & Barker, M. J. (eds.). *The Palgrave handbook of the psychology of sexuality and gender* (pp. 60–76). London: Palgrave-Macmillan.

(2017). [Monograph]. *Trans and sexuality – An existentially-informed ethical enquiry with implications for counselling psychology.* London: Routledge.

Richards, C., & Barker. M. (2013). *Sexuality and gender for mental health professionals: A practical guide.* London: Sage.

Richards, C., Farndon, H., Gibson, S., Jamieson, R., Moon, I., Lenihan, P., Rimes, K., & Semlyen, J. (2019). *Guidelines for psychologists working with gender, sexuality and relationship diversity* (2nd ed.). London: British Psychological Society.

White, T., & Ettner, R. (2007). Adaptation and adjustment in children of transsexual parents. *European Child & Adolescent Psychiatry, 16*(4), 215–221.

World Health Organization. (2019a). 6D36 Paraphilic disorder involving solitary behaviour or consenting individuals. In *WHO International statistical classification of diseases and related health problems 11.* Geneva: WHO.

World Health Organization. (2019b). *International statistical classification of diseases and related health problems 11.* Geneva: WHO.

Chapter 9

Legal and Religious Aspects

Introduction

The legal aspects of a change of social gender role are important, if for no other reason than the law matters a lot. Sadly in some countries, there is no possibility of a change of legal gender; indeed, there can be appalling prohibitions against it. In others, there is a very limited and onerous set of options. Consequently this chapter will focus upon the UK legal system, as a discussion of all of the varied global legislation associated with gender would be a book in its own right, although interested readers may wish to read the excellent work of the International Lesbian Gay Bisexual, Trans and Intersex Association (ILGA.org) for further detail on this.

This discussion of the pertinence of a legal as well as social change of gender is important if in later life, a person should want to acquire legal recognition of their gender via a Gender Recognition Certificate afforded by (at the time of writing) the Gender Recognition Act (HMSO, 2004) or forthcoming legislation, a lot of weight will be placed on when, exactly, that person made a formal, legal, change of name. The Gender Recognition Panel that issues such certificates is a branch of the judiciary and as lawyers they, unsurprisingly, care about the law.

Legal issues also matter particularly for young trans folk who are living at home with parents who are not particularly understanding or supportive, not for legal reasons as such but rather because such young people find themselves trapped in 'the liminal zone'. A liminal zone can be physical, age related, geographical, seasonal, or whatever. Put simply, it is a place where the usual social rules somehow don't apply. For example, if one is a student at the University of Thetley-on-Thames studying biochemistry and it is unseasonably hot weather, it is considered to be a slightly wacky, studenty thing to do to turn up at lectures in a pair of pyjamas. "Young people, eh! What wacky things they do!" is likely to be the response. It is worthwhile noting that somehow it would not be all right for the biochemistry lecturer to turn up in a pair of pyjamas even though she's at the same university and in the same lecture and is just as overheated. Clearly, different sorts of rules apply to the students simply because they are young. In this case, youth itself has operated as a liminal zone.

The liminal zone of youth confers advantage in that young people can be cut a considerable amount of slack. The difficulty, on the other hand, is that the same liminal zone effect means that young people tend not to be taken seriously. A 17-year-old can have a brilliant idea and when announcing it to the world receive as a response "young people, eh! What wacky ideas they have!" If precisely the same idea is generated and expressed by somebody age 30, he is likely instead to be given an enterprise award and a government department to run and widely hailed as an innovative business guru.

This liminal zone effect is particularly marked in a family setting. It is exceedingly difficult for younger people to be taken seriously by people who, not so very many years earlier, were wiping their bottoms and spooning food down their tiny mouths. The problem becomes even more acute when the feelings are surprising or unwelcome, such as a desire to change social gender role might be.

How can younger people break out of the liminal zone? What is required is a strategy that is faster than just waiting until they are old enough not to be 'young' any more. In these trying circumstances, it is amazing what a difference legal documents make. By way of example, consider the following thought experiment.

Imagine someone named John, age 18 years and 3 days, enthusing to his parents about his girlfriend, Tracey, who goes to the same college and is the same age. He might assure them that theirs is a love that will never die and that they will be together forever. Doubtless, his parents would agree that she seems a really nice girl and in a rather tepid way wish them both the best of luck before returning to drinking a mug of cocoa and watching *Antiques Roadshow* on the TV.

Now imagine that the next day, in the course of the lunch break at college, John and Tracey pop up to the town centre and get married in the registry office. They are both older than 18 and so are perfectly legally entitled to do this.

That evening, if John were to inform his parents that he married Tracey in the lunch break, one imagines that they would sit bolt upright and pay a whole lot more attention to the situation than they did the day before. Why is this? John and Tracey feel exactly the same way about each other as they did the day before, after all.

What is different, of course, is that they have legally married. This has become a relationship which has legal recognition outside the family and friend environment. The wider administrative structures of society will view them differently. John's parents will be compelled, of course, to view Tracey differently – as a daughter-in-law, for a start.

Consequently, it is particularly important for people who have made a clear decision regarding their gender and have established it in the wider world, to continue this by making a clear and legal statement by changing their name, re-registering in their new name and new gender role in the many places where we are all registered, and to acquire the associated documentation. It is a good first step which renders subsequent steps easier to accomplish and less likely to provoke resistance from family, institutions, and potentially awkward individuals. Naturally we are not discussing people for whom a legal change is not yet fully possible, including non-binary people, whom we will discuss later, or people who do not have the wherewithal to make such a change (see Chapter 6, *Forensic Settings*). For now, suffice it to say that such change as is possible will likely bring benefits when it is made.

A useful additional step to this establishing oneself in the wider world relating to younger people is that of insisting on paying rent, of some amount, to their parents. It doesn't matter if they are financially dependent on those very same people; there is nonetheless something symbolic and significant about paying rent for the following reasons:

First, it encourages the person to think of their parents more as landlords. Nobody expects or feels that their landlord can decide how they should live their lives.

Second, it encourages the parents to think of the young person as more of a tenant and less of a child. Tenants are expected to behave in a civil way, keep the common areas of the house tidy and so forth but otherwise are free to live as they will.

Third (and this is something which hopefully will not be needed) as a tenant, the young person can't be thrown out of the house just like that. The landlords (the parents) need to give any tenant (in this case the young person) three months' notice. If there is a dramatic scene ending up with "Get out of our house!" the young person doesn't have to go. If there are threats to "call the police to throw you out" and the police are actually called, they will agree that amateurish though the tenancy arrangement looks, nonetheless tenancy agreement it is. And three months is just enough time for the young person to secure another place to live. Those young people who are under age 25 and in the United Kingdom are eligible for help from the excellent Albert Kennedy Trust (www.akt.org.uk), which offers housing advice and help for LGBT folk under age 25 who have been thrown out or otherwise rendered homeless.

The Law

Changing of Name

In the United Kingdom, a change of name is easily done and carries enormous legal, symbolic, and emotional significance. Achieving this in a formal, official way is particularly important because common, customary nicknames just aren't the same, no matter how widely they are used. For this reason, the onerous processes in place in some other countries can unnecessarily disadvantage trans people (and others), and it is noticeable how few problems the simple UK system creates, and indeed how many other judicial systems are in the process of having a similar more easily accessed arrangement.

In the United Kingdom, the obvious first step in changing one's name is to think of what to change it to. In considering this, it's worthwhile thinking of what functions a name carries. Clearly, it encapsulates something of one's own identity, but it also serves as information to transmit to others, sometimes the only information they have in advance of an arrival in person. A maladroit choice risks unwelcome scrutiny, incongruity, or ambiguity. Indeed, it is not uncommon for some younger people to choose a name which resonates, perhaps from a contemporary media source such as graphic novels, film, computer games, anime, and the like, which upon maturing no longer seems appropriate.

It can also be worthwhile considering what name might have been given had the person been assigned to the correct gender at birth. For example, it is extremely unlikely that somebody born in 1972 would have been called "Chelsea". In 1972, Chelsea was a district of London or a football team. It wasn't commonly thought of as anybody's name until US President Bill Clinton applied it to his daughter, after which it became frequently used in this way. If somebody born prior to 1972 were to change their name to "Chelsea", it more or less advertises that they have changed their name at some point. This might be a problem, or it might not. It is, at least, worthwhile for the trans person to be aware of this.

In a related vein, it is somewhat bold to make a change to something which is an abbreviation of a longer name. Parents do not generally name their children "Mick", "Bob", or "Dave". Rather, they name them Michael, Robert, or David, and their children are known in later life by those nicknames. If the trans person chooses "Mick", "Bob", or "Dave" as an actual, legal first name, it might give the impression that either they had relaxed parents or, alternatively, they have changed their name. Both might, or might not, be what is intended.

Lastly, there may be problems associated with a name which is not immediately apprehended by others as being either that of a man or of a woman. This is ideal for a non-binary person, of course, but non-binary names for men or women may leave others uncertain as to what the gender is of the person about to walk in the door and consequently leave them scrutinising rather more closely than a binary trans person might wish.

For binary trans people, an unambiguous name tells people in advance what they should expect. On the whole, people have a tendency to apprehend what they are expecting to see – which should be exactly what the trans person wants them to. Even if, on closer inspection, they guess that the person in front of them has changed gender role, an unambiguous name at the very least gives them a clear suggestion of how the person in front of them ought to be treated. Usefully, the increasing prominence of trans folk in the broadcast media leaves the great general public thinking (admittedly usually wrongly) they know a bit about it all; consequently, they are fairly likely to think "blimey, it's one of those transsexual people like I've seen on the TV" and have at least the idea that they should not make a fuss and treat the person as their name indicates they wish to be treated. Those who are prejudiced are correspondingly less likely to give expression to their views because they have the feeling that it's no longer socially acceptable to do so in the same way that homophobia isn't acceptable any more, vaguely feeling that it might now be illegal in some sort of way that they aren't sure of (outright prejudice is, of course, illegal under the Equality Act (HMSO, 2010)) and which is, they privately think, yet another sign of everything going to hell in a handcart.

A change of name in the United Kingdom is not expensive. For people born in the United Kingdom with straightforward British citizenship, older than age 18, the necessary form can be downloaded from the internet for free. It needs to be witnessed by two people who are not family members, who are older than age 18, British citizens, and mentally competent. The witnesses don't have to be solicitors, doctors, or other similarly exalted people. The trans person needs to be reminded to make sure that they don't sign the document *before* the witnesses see it and to make sure that they are both present at the same time to personally observe any signature. An alternative is to secure the services of a solicitor, which can have a pleasing sense of ceremony, and which may be beneficial in more complex cases but is usually unnecessary.

Once a change of name deed or statutory declaration has been completed, there follows the rather more tedious and exhausting work of re-registering the new name and with a new sex marker in all the very many places where we are all registered. These would include the bank, primary care, dentist, any clubs or societies, student loan company, college, university, job, benefits agency, probation officer, council tax, library, electoral roll, and on and on and on. Generally it takes about a year to change absolutely all the registrations, as there are some institutions that do not communicate any more frequently than annually.

Changing a Title

The prefix Miss, Ms, Mx, Mr, Master, or Mrs put in front of names is frequently described in computer drop-down forms as a "title". In point of fact, a title is something which denotes rank, privilege, or training (professor, admiral, doctor would be examples). Miss, Mx, Ms, Mr, Master, and Mrs are not actually ranks and require no training to achieve. Consequently, in law they are termed *styles of address* and don't carry any particular force. It's a bit like men appending *Esquire* behind a name – it looks rather grand but means nothing at all, and anyone can do it. What follows from this is that anyone may change their style of address from the masculine Mr to the more feminine Miss, Ms, or even

Mrs, or do the reverse, exactly as they wish. Happily, increasing numbers of places will allow a change to a gender-neutral style of address such as Mx. While this is excellent news for non-binary people who prefer it, a non-binary style of address isn't a good idea if non-binary is not what is sought. It can sometimes, oddly, be strongly suggested by institutions for use by binary trans people – that is trans men or trans women – however, if a non-binary gender is not the aim the person should push for the style of address that is wanted and appropriate and not settle for anything less. Certainly in health settings, the patient should be gendered in almost all cases precisely as they prefer – whether binary or not (see Chapter 5, *Supporting Trans and Non-binary People in Mental Health Services*, for the rare exceptions to this).

Changing Registrations

Nearly all institutions will readily make changes upon sight of a change of name deed. Usually, registration numbers such as banking details will remain unchanged. In the United Kingdom, people changing gender role have the option of changing their National Health Service number and National Insurance number, also. Whether it's wise to exercise that right is debatable. Changing a National Insurance number raises the worrying possibility of losing administrative access to accrued National Insurance money. This could be a problem in the event of a benefits payment failure because it might well be that the only person in the Benefits Agency office senior enough to be able to put the matter right is on a week's training course in Darlington.

Changing a National Health Service number will mean that any admitting medical team will be unable to find out anything about the medical history, allergies, previous immunisations, and the like. Health problems might result. In addition, if a patient changes their NHS number while undergoing treatment for gender dysphoria, the records of those treatments will be registered to the new number, making the exercise of debatable utility in terms of 'hiding' one's trans status. Notwithstanding this, there is, of course, an argument for having an NHS number which accords with one's identity.

Banks seem to vary so much in their requirements for changing name and sex marker on their accounts that the only plausible explanation is that no universal rule applies even within any one bank, let alone one accepted by all of them. What must be avoided at all costs, though, is trying to open a bank account with a document that has the wrong sex marker and cannot be changed, like some sorts of non-UK passports. If the trans person is a non-UK passport holder with a nationality that doesn't make such changes easy (or even, in some cases, possible), it would be wise to try to instead use other documents. It is possible to open a bank account without a passport, of course, as do the thousands of people who have a bank account but have never travelled abroad. If a bank is being really difficult, it might be easier to simply open a whole new bank account, with the right details, with another bank and then just transfer all banking affairs from the old bank to the new one before closing the old account.

Occasionally, institutions assert that such changes aren't possible unless the trans person has a Gender Recognition Certificate (see later discussion). This is entirely false. The only personal identity records which cannot be changed without the possession of a Gender Recognition Certificate are those with the Pensions Agency and the birth certificate.

Changing Existing Exam Certificates

Examination certificates, diplomas, degree certificates, and similar documents can often be changed to the new name, retrospectively. Examination of the crest in the middle of the document reveals which authority awarded the qualification. This is not the school attended but rather the examination board which set the exam, marked it, and printed the certificate. Awarding authorities will often give new certificates with the new name, provided the person can give the old ones back, sometimes charging a small fee for doing so. It can be more awkward if there are no old certificates. If the original certificate proudly records attendance at a boy's or girl's school, this detail can be removed on the new certificate.

It can be worthwhile changing secondary school examination certificates in this way even if people have substantial higher qualifications because emigration to many English-speaking foreign countries requires migrants to produce documentary evidence that they are competent in the English language. Simply coming from another English-speaking country isn't considered adequate (there are, after all, many people in England who possess a UK passport but can't speak English) and GCSE English answers that requirement rather nicely.

Changing a Passport and Driving Licence

A passport and driving licence are particularly important documents to change to a new name and sex marker, not simply because they entitle the bearer to drive a car or travel abroad (although they are very handy in that regard) but also because they represent photographic identification of the sort frequently insisted on by banks and some governmental departments. Of the two, probably the most useful and certainly the cheapest to obtain is a driving licence. It is a convenient size, made of durable plastic, and unlikely to be stolen, in part because just about everybody can easily get one, which is more than can be said for a British passport. If a passport is accidentally put through the laundry, the result is paper maché. Do the same with a driving licence and all that results is a literally clean licence. Trans people may be reminded that owning a *provisional* driving licence in no way obliges them to attempt to learn to drive, a skill which is an expensive and perhaps obsolescent achievement in many cases, what with the self-driving car being imminent and increasing numbers of people living in cities with mass transportation and congested roads. For these purposes, the provisional licence is best thought of as a form of identity card.

The Driver and Vehicle Licensing Authority and the Passport Agency will change a name on receipt of a statutory declaration but may require confirmation of a permanent and full-time change of social gender role from a medical professional or applied psychologist to change a sex marker. In the case of the driving licence, one digit in the fifth line on the licence (the driver number) will change from a zero or a one into a five or a six to denote a change of sex from male to female (or the reverse). Sadly gender-neutral ID documents are not yet available, although sensible arguments are being made that they should be, as generally the gender of the person driving the car or travelling abroad is not relevant, or no more relevant than other characteristics which are not thought necessary to record on these documents.

Obtaining a Citizen's Card

If a trans person is unable to obtain a driver's licence because of a physical condition such as poor eyesight or epilepsy, for example, a reasonable substitute can be a Citizen's Card. Legislation to introduce these was passed by Prime Minister Tony Blair's administration, but the cards proved unpopular and take-up was low. Nonetheless, the legislation enabling people to get one still exists and the cards are still perfectly obtainable and widely accepted, particularly by governmental organisations which are obliged to accept them as they are government issued in the first place.

Trans Person Not a UK Passport Holder?

For non-UK passport holders, the mechanism to change the name or sex marker on the passport will be what applies in the jurisdiction which issued that passport. Many countries will allow a change of name fairly easily, but a change of sex marker can be much harder or, sometimes, impossible. Many countries allow this in theory but have legislation of Byzantine complexity or with such Draconian conditions needed to achieve it that it can actually sometimes be less emotionally taxing and financially draining for the trans person to apply for UK citizenship, if eligible. It's worthwhile bearing in mind that non-UK citizenship does not affect anyone applying for a driving licence and that such a licence can be used in combination with proof of address (such as a utility bill) for most identification purposes.

Obtaining a Gender Recognition Certificate

A UK Gender Recognition Certificate (GRC) is a document awarded by the Gender Recognition Panel (GRP), a branch of the Appeals Directorate of the Judiciary. To gain a certificate, one has to have lived for two years in one's gender role, usually taken from the date of the change of name (see earlier discussion) and have two reports prepared, one from a clinician recognised by HM Courts and Tribunals Service as a specialist in the field of Gender Dysphoria. There is no requirement to have physical changes, the reasoning being an understandable distaste for state-mandated sterilization for bureaucratic reasons, as well as a reluctance to ask people to risk incontinence, loss of sexual function, and other surgical and hormonal risks for them to have their gender legally recognised.

The GRC acts to retrospectively change legal sex to one other than that assigned at birth but unfortunately cannot, at the time of writing, denote non-binary gender status. In effect, the law considers the recipient to be the new sex and to have always been so, save with regard to some aspects of previous crimes and to parenthood. This latter is subject to challenge, for example, if a trans man has given birth to children, he will remain the mother of those children even though if he were to adopt other children, he would be those children's father. Upon receipt of a GRC, any trans person born in the United Kingdom can be provided with a new birth certificate which will show the new name and new sex. Do note, however, that it is the GRC and not the birth certificate which confers the legal gender.

In practice, only limited practical change automatically results from the acquisition of a Gender Recognition Certificate. Birth certificates are not readily accepted as a means of identification by government institutions, banks, and the like, all of which generally want to see photographic identification such as a passport or driving licence. Financial matters will remain unaltered, also, save for those pensions and entitlements which vary with sex, of which there are increasingly few. For these, a change of legal sex could act to advantage or could be disadvantageous; it's worthwhile to work out the consequences in advance, since the process can't be reversed even if they have inadvertently ended up in a position where they are going to have to work for five more years before claiming a pension, or if they will be rendered unable to claim on a spouse's pension.

One unfortunate and unintended consequence of obtaining a Gender Recognition Certificate can be a change in liability to inherit property left in a will:

- If the name in the will is the old ('dead') name and the date on the will is before the Gender Recognition Certificate was issued, the trans person will be unaffected.

- If the name in the will is the new name and the date on the will is after the awarding of a Gender Recognition Certificate, the trans person will be unaffected as well.
- The problem comes if the name on the will is the old name and the date on the will is after the Gender Recognition Certificate was awarded. In this situation, the trans person, as named in the will, doesn't exist at all and never did – and so cannot inherit. It could be worthwhile, in financial terms if no other, for the trans person to alert those writing or amending a will of this potential pitfall.

Having said that there are few practical benefits, there can be, for some, a significant personal benefit in having one's gender unequivocally recognised by the State. No matter what some bloke down the pub may think – the entire State begs to differ, so to speak.

We should note here that one cannot generally ask a trans person for a GRC as proof of gender when going about their lawful business – using a toilet or dressing room or being admitted to hospital, for example (see later discussion) – the law specifically does not allow a person to be forced to prove their gender in this way.

Disclosure by a Health Professional That a Person is Trans

The Gender Recognition Act (HMSO, 2004) and The Gender Recognition (Disclosure of Information) (England, Wales and Northern Ireland) Order 2005 (HMSO, 2005) make it a criminal offence to disclose that a person is trans if that information is collected in the course of one's professional role and the trans person has not given consent to such disclosure. Note that this is a *criminal* offence – it is not that one would be sued by the patient (although that may follow), but that one would be arrested, charged, convicted, and fined or given a prison sentence and have a criminal record – things which are frowned upon by statutory healthcare regulators such as the GMC and the HCPC. And then they are likely to be sued. It is also an absolute offence – there are no 'reasonableness criteria' for dictation, supervision, letters to GPs or the like; one cannot say "we always do … " "the system is set up … " "trust policy is that … " or any other such thing. The law overrides all these considerations. Very simply one must ask the patient for consent to disclose. This must legally be a limited disclosure to a certain set of people or professionals. The only exception to this is when the patient is unable to consent through lack of capacity *on this matter* and the detailed specifications for these very specific circumstances are laid down in The Gender Recognition (Disclosure of Information) (England, Wales and Northern Ireland) Order 2005 (HMSO, 2005).

The simplest way to ask patients to disclose is to add it into one's usual consenting and administrative procedures. Of course, it should be given to everyone and not just those people one suspects of 'looking trans', as inevitably other trans people will be missed and some cisgender people will be confused.

Getting Married

Since the adoption of The Marriage (Same Sex Couples) Act 2013 in the United Kingdom, there has been no requirement for trans people to obtain a Gender Recognition Certificate to get married. If they do not obtain a certificate, though, the form of words used in the ceremony would be that for a same-sex couple if a trans man were marrying a cisgender woman or a trans woman were marrying a cisgender man. In a related way, same-gender marriages where one partner is a trans person will require the use of the different-gender couple form of words in the ceremony. This incongruity can only be legally avoided if the trans person obtains a Gender Recognition Certificate.

If the Registrar were to fail to apprehend that one of the prospective couple was a trans person, and if the trans person were to fail to enlighten the Registrar, the marriage would go ahead using an incorrect form of words. If such a matter were to come to legal attention later, the marriage would probably not be "void" (a circumstance where the court is obliged to cancel the marriage) but rather would be "voidable" (a circumstance where the court is empowered to cancel the marriage but isn't obliged to do so). The reaction of a court in this circumstance has yet to be tested. This is important as there is not yet legal equality between same-sex and different-sex marriages in terms of pension rights and so on, and not yet equality between marriage (of any sort) and civil partnerships.

Avoiding Unintentionally Outing Yourself with a DBS Check

Many jobs in the United Kingdom, both paid and voluntary, require applicants to submit an application to the Disclosures and Barring Service. These 'DBS checks' (or 'CRB checks' as they are often still sometimes spoken of) routinely ask whether there has been a change of name and, if this is so, what name applied before. People applying for a job who don't want to disclose an earlier change of gender role – perhaps because they are 'in stealth' – are entitled to fill in the form as if they have never changed their name if they additionally contact the Sensitive Applications Team at the Disclosures and Barring Service. This service will intercept the application in DBS offices and tell the employer all about the relevant criminal convictions but disclose nothing about the change of gender role; the law holds that a change of gender role could never be a reason for an employer to have a problem and as a consequence there's never a reason for them to know.

Medical Records

Medical records are a special case to the general rule that one should treat people as their experienced gender. This is because the records relate to certain bodily parts and functions which are most commonly associated with one sex. Nonetheless, people should be treated holistically and should not be assumed to be 'really' of their birth-assigned gender. Old names and styles of address should not generally be used. Irrelevant information regarding gender should not be recorded. The best approach is simply to append a note about the specific circumstances where it is pertinent – for example, if a trans woman has not had feminising hormonal treatment, her blood results will be measured against 'male' ranges. Simply noting that this should be so and that the female range from the labs needs reinterpreting is all that is required.

When a person makes a formal change of gender role, discussions should be had as to the advantages and disadvantages of sealing the old records – bearing in mind that the Gender Recognition Act will apply here.

Non-binary Matters

People who identify as neither male nor female – non-binary people – are in the unenviable position of not having their gender legally recognised. This is unfortunate as gender is still so common in so much of the bureaucratic machinery of everyday life. Moves are afoot to change this, with increasing numbers of jurisdictions cutting down on unnecessary requests to state gender, and the options to use Mx styles of address on ID documents or X markers on passports instead of M or F. At present in the United Kingdom, it is not possible to update a passport or driving licence, but ad hoc arrangements are common. For example, people may update bank cards, utility bills, and so on with Mx and their gender-neutral name. Doubtless governmental policy and law will reflect this soon, although there are forensic considerations which must be resolved first (see Chapter 6, *Forensic Settings*). Health professionals should strive to accommodate non-binary people within their systems, only making recourse to legal gender when it is absolutely necessary.

Toilets!

The British seem to have an ability, unsurpassed in all Europe, to get themselves steamed up about trans folk and toilets. In France and Germany, unisex toilets are unremarkable features and one has to travel all the way to the Southeast of the United States to find anywhere where quite so much emotional heat is generated by the issue of where, exactly, bodily wastes should be evacuated.

The matter is really rather simple: essentially, if someone is living as a woman, she should be using the women's toilet (and let's be honest there is never a furore about 'women' in men's toilets). To do otherwise simply confuses others and makes the trans woman feel diminished and humiliated. The worry, of course, is that someone will "make a fuss" in a public toilet, tell her that she can't use it, or threaten to call the police. If this does happen (and it's not at all common), it's worthwhile noting that the kind of person who wants to make an issue over this sort of thing is, happily, also the kind of person who tends to be impressed by formal, legal documents. While having to present documents should never be necessary in this situation, having an appropriate sex marker and name on her passport and driving licence usually silences people like this, leaving them with the vague and unsettling sense that maybe it is they who have broken the law in some way (who are they to argue with the Passport Agency and Driver and Vehicle Licensing Authority, after all?).

Sometimes things do go so far as threats to 'call the police'. If called, the police will arrive – they are very good that way – but their response when they arrive will, in the vast majority of cases, be the same as it should be if they were called because someone wanted to complain that there was a black person in the toilet. They advise the caller to stop making a fuss, in the first instance. If the fuss continues, they advise the upset person to seek another, more commodious toilet that might suit them better. If both these measures fail, they take action, but this should never be against the trans person; it is the continued fuss which constitutes a breach of the peace.

The key issue in toilets isn't which toilet is used but how people conduct themselves in the toilet. Anyone who calmly goes about the business of evacuating their bodily wastes in the conventional manner is acceptable. Personal bodily constitution can never be objected to, only behaviour – and that is not pertinent only to trans people. If someone is behaving in an untoward way in a toilet, they will be arrested or sectioned – whether they are trans or cisgender. As a rule, trans people just wish to go about their lives and are perhaps therefore *less* likely to behave in an untoward way.

A slightly different variation on this theme occurs if there is a change in gender role in the setting of a workplace, college, or university. It is sometimes wrongly stated that the trans person should be "using the disabled toilet". That this is inappropriate can usually be made clear by a (rather tongue in cheek) request to use the disabled parking spot being refused. Sometimes there is the even more bizarre suggestion that a requirement is having had some sort of genital surgery, but this can usually be rebutted by acceptance on condition of the suggested genital inspection applying to all other employees as well.

One solution to this is the increasing availability of gender-neutral toilets. Accessible toilets have long been gender neutral, as have the toilets in many smaller restaurants and cafés for example – seldom with any difficulties.[1] Such facilities also allow non-binary people less stressful access to this most basic of human facilities.

Sports – Competing after a Change of Gender Role

In practice, things vary greatly from sport to sport and each governing body makes its own rules. There are even some sports, boxing and cheerleading are examples, where there are two governing bodies rather than one, and their rules on trans folk don't always agree – a cheerleading squad with a trans woman would be able to deploy her in competitions under one code but not the other, for example.

Most sports set much store on testosterone levels – the assumption that the higher testosterone levels seen in trans men on treatment or in trans women without testicular suppression will confer an advantage. It seems to be thought that if a trans woman has a testosterone level in the 'normal female range' (such a range is itself a matter of dispute), she can fairly compete with cisgender women (actually, she might be working at a disadvantage if her muscle strength has been reduced to that expected in a cisgender woman of her height because those possibly slightly more feeble muscles will all still be attached to her rather heavier 'cisgender man's' skeleton). It seems often to be assumed that if a trans woman's testes have been removed or their function stopped with a gonadotrophin-releasing hormone analogue at least two years earlier, there won't be a problem.

All that being said, in those sports where men and women are able to compete together, it is by no means assured that men will always win[2] – meaning trans women without suppressed testosterone would not necessarily win either. It is notable how, as more women are entering sports, and as physical strength becomes more acceptable for [cisgender] women, the gaps are closing. Some sports which rely on reach separate by gender on the basis that a man's longer reach would put women at a disadvantage, but without considering that it puts shorter men at a disadvantage. Perhaps separation based on reach in such sports, rather than gender, might be an option in such cases. Certainly more research remains to be undertaken, and doubtless shifting cultural norms will play a part.

Religion

Trans and God – the Relationship with Religions and with Faith

Although the obligations and prohibitions found in religions are not the law of the land, for many trans people, and more often for the families of trans people, they may be just as

---

[1] Except perhaps the need for strict segregation between the Messy and the Clean – sprinklers and hoverers we are considering you here.

[2] See rock climber Lynne Hill's first free ascent of the Nose on El Capitan and Jasmin Paris's record for the 268-mile Spine [running] Race, for example.

important or even more so. Religiousness and particularly 'religious fundamentalism' seem more prominent now than in many previous decades. Where once there was widespread cooperation between sects within a faith group and sometimes even open and frank cooperation between faith groups, fostered perhaps by a common perception of an increasingly secular world, there seems now to be competition or even hostility. As the various faith groups have grown more proactive and strident, each has formulated a doctrinal view on an increasing number of aspects of the contemporary world including, of course, a view on trans folk. The position of some of the major faith groups is summarised in the following sections.

The Jewish View

Jewish law contains 613 commandments and prohibitions of which only a few seem pertinent to trans folk. The first is detailed in Deuteronomy 22:5, which says "there will not be a man's implement on a woman, and a man will not put on a woman's dress, because it is an abomination before HASHEM your G-d all who do these." The second is that it is forbidden for male Jews to castrate themselves.

It is, however, accepted that violation of some laws is acceptable if life is saved thereby: "better to violate one Shabat so that he will be able to observe many Shabbatot" even if the violation is lifelong (as in the consumption of life-preserving drugs containing proscribed things).

Rabbi Eliezer Waldenberg is considered the pre-eminent religious legal authority in Israel and in most sites outside the United States (where Rabbi Moshe Feinstein is favoured). He is thought to have particular authority in medical matters. He is the only (or only major) religious authority to have addressed the question of trans folk.

Rabbi Waldenberg maintained that the external genital organs, as visible to the naked eye, were the determinants of sexual status in Jewish law, and working from this premise made a judgement in the case of androgen insensitivity syndrome. Androgen insensitivity syndrome is the congenital lack of testosterone receptors in someone with XY chromosomes. He noted that oestrogen therapy renders male testes non-functional and casts doubt over whether removing such non-functional organs amounts to castration. He noted also that the testes are rendered non-functional by degrees as oestrogens are given, implying a lack of a single castrating act. This might render the non-functionality as having arisen from a cause other than a castration.

Rabbi Waldenberg noted that in genital reconstructive surgery, if it happens at all, patients do not castrate themselves; the surgeon does it. The question instead becomes whether Jewish trans women undergoing genital reconstructive surgery have been guilty of the violation of causing another (the surgeon) to transgress. It is not clear whether this would be applicable if the surgeon were anything other than another Jewish person.

Regarding clothing, the Rabbi noted that a lifetime of cross-dressing without genital surgery would represent a greater violation than a more limited one. Of cross-dressing as part of a treatment programme followed by genital reconstructive surgery, it was reasoned that since the latter would render the person female, such dressing is thus no longer a violation. This would be a circumstance in which a shorter violation is acceptable to prevent a longer-term violation.

Lastly, the Rabbi noted that preventing trans folk from having either genital surgery or cross-dressing would, while preventing the clear violation of prolonged cross-dressing and the violation of self-castration (if his early arguments were not accepted), have a high chance of death from suicide. He invoked the preservation of life as an accepted reason to break the Sabbath rules.

The Mainstream Church of England View

The mainstream Church of England does not have a fixed doctrinal position on trans folk. It should be noted, though, that ordained Church of England priests have changed their gender role and have remained in their occupation. This is not necessarily well accepted by the evangelical wing of the Church of England, and it seems fair to say that the Church of England contains within it a multiplicity of opinions and manages to contain these by having no rigid doctrinal position.

The Jehovah's Witness View

This faith group has a doctrinally based objection to both the change of gender role and genital reconstructive surgery, particularly when the change is from male to female. It is maintained that people who wear clothing of 'another' gender and those who have undergone genital surgery cannot become Jehovah's Witnesses, even if they have legally changed their gender marker, unless they are willing to take the painful step of reverting to their original gender role. It is believed that while clinical reversal is not possible, lifestyle reversal is. The sole exceptions to this are those people who were born with both male and female genital organs, and it is the responsibility of the individual to prove that this is the case.

Particularly observant Jehovah's Witnesses will "disfellowship" from their faith group anyone who has changed social gender role. This involves a total lack of communication by all other Witnesses, including family members and closest friends.

The Roman Catholic View

The Roman Catholic Church is opposed to any attempt by someone whose physical characteristics are unambiguously of one sex to have those characteristics altered so as to resemble those of the other sex. Whilst it recognises the suffering caused by gender dysphoria, it does not believe that surgery or the use of hormones is the answer to that suffering. It is maintained that those who are (at least physically) healthy should not be 'mutilated' by surgical procedures: the belief is that trans people should be encouraged, as far as possible, to fit their self-perception to their bodies.

That being said, it is held also that the Church is the refuge of sinners and in practical terms no particular opposition appears to follow; less formal guidance adhered to by many suggests that where there is a conflict between doctrine and compassion, compassion should be the route followed.

The Evangelical Christian View

Whilst recognising that all of us are sinners and maintaining that the only real hope for sinful people, of every sexual orientation and gender identity, is for wholeness that is to be found only in Jesus Christ – it is maintained that God created human beings as either male or female and that an authentic change from anyone's given sex is both impossible and incompatible with God's will as revealed in Scripture and in creation. It is maintained by this group that acceptance of the gospel of Jesus Christ affords opportunities for holistic change in the context of non-surgical solutions. Any hurt caused to trans folk by unwelcoming or rejecting attitudes on the part of the church is rejected and congregations are called upon to welcome and accept trans folk, whilst acknowledging the need for parallel teaching and discernment, particularly where children are concerned. It is hoped and anticipated that trans folk will come in due course to accede to the need to reorient their lifestyle in accordance with this understanding of biblical principles and orthodox church teaching.

The Buddhist View

There seems to be no single view in Buddhism, an ancient faith having its origins in northern India, subsequently spreading throughout much of Asia and then globally. Often, it seems, what may appear as a Buddhist attitude may be more indicative of the culture within which it is expressed. Buddhists are often accepting of monks and nuns who show cross-gendered behaviour staying in their holy orders, along with those of their new gender, and follow their respective codes of conduct. In Western Buddhist thought, the belief is that basic Buddhist principles are just as relevant to trans folk as to anyone else and that tolerance and kindness are the most appropriate responses.

The Hindu View

This faith maintains that gender identity is temporary, as is the material body, since one's gender identity can change from lifetime to lifetime. It is held that physical or psychological gender identity is very separate and different from spiritual or eternal identity. Religious texts describe male, female, and a third gender, seeming to include asexual people, people with diversity of sexual characteristics, same-sex-attracted people, and trans folk. This faith group maintains that the gates of the spiritual world are just as open for third-gender people as they are for anyone else and that discrimination against those of a third gender is contradictory to the Hindu theology.

The Islamic View

The only clear, public statement about trans folk and genital reconstructive surgery in an Islamic context dates from 1987. An Iranian trans woman was introduced via an intermediary Islamic scholar, from whom she had sought advice, to Ayatollah Khomeni. The Ayatollah was at that time a noted Shia Islamic scholar living in Iraq. He judged that she needed a clear sexual identity to carry out her religious duties and that accordingly later genital reconstructive surgery would be acceptable. In later life, he became the leader of modern revolutionary Iran and where a change of social gender role and subsequent genital reconstructive surgery are legal. This being said, it seems that Iranian social acceptance has not entirely followed from legal acceptability and that ordinary life in Iran for trans folk is still very difficult.

What Is God Saying to This Person?

There is a clear distinction to be made between the doctrines of the faith group into which any trans person was born, the religious doctrines in which they personally believe, and the direct communication between them and God.

If the trans person's experience conflicts with the faith group into which they were born, and they have not themselves any particular religious faith, they may experience excommunication from the faith group, otherwise supportive though it may have been. They may then find themselves in the position of having to garner a new and supportive social circle.

If, instead, they have a genuine religious faith, the most important question, surely, must be whether they feel God is troubled by a change of social gender role on their part. If their communication with God, howsoever it is achieved, indicates to them that there is no disapproval from the deity, then this must be more important than what any doctrinal group or faith thinks or maintains, since all written doctrines, outpourings from the fountain of God as they may be, cannot be the fountain in and of themselves. Trans people who have a secure relationship with God but experience rejection from their faith group are in a much stronger position than the other way around. It may be that another sect within the same faith group may be more accepting.

Summary

Legal matters affect trans people in terms of both access to services and other people's acceptance that people are indeed who they say they are. On a human level, this is unfortunate, as the law should act at the far ends of decent human experience, not be the start of it.[3] Trans people should be treated decently, and as being of their gender – whether binary or non-binary – irrespective of their current legal situation, or what the law provides. When recourse to law is absolutely necessary, it should be done in a context of understanding, compassion, and respect for the rights of the individual.

Further Reading

Campbell, M., Hinton, J. D., & Anderson, J. R. (2019). A systematic review of the relationship between religion and attitudes toward transgender and gender-variant people. *International Journal of Transgenderism, 20*(1), 21–38.

Clucas, R., & Whittle, S. (2018). Law. In C. Richards., W. P. Bouman., & M. J. Barker (eds.), *Genderqueer and non-binary genders* (pp. 73–99). London: Palgrave-Macmillan.

International Lesbian Gay Bisexual, Trans and Intersex Association – ILGA.org

The Yogyakarta Principles. (2007). *The Yogyakarta Principles on the application of international human rights law in relation to sexual orientation and gender identity.* Available at www.yogyakartaprinciples.org/principles_en.pdf

References

HMSO. (2004). Gender Recognition Act.

HMSO. (2005). The Gender Recognition (Disclosure of Information) (England, Wales and Northern Ireland) Order 2005.

HMSO. (2010). The Equality Act.

---

[3] As a metaphor consider that while it is absolutely right that we do not sleep with our patients, we do not see what we can get away with within the bounds of the law. The law is the far edge, not our everyday guideline.

Psychotherapy

Introduction

Psychotherapy with gender diverse people will proceed much as with cisgender people and for the same range of issues – be it bereavement, job issues, childhood trauma, relationship issues, mood disorders, psychosis, personality difficulties, and so on – although with the usual mannered inflection[1] one would expect for any form of diversity. The usual principles of establishing good rapport and then utilising the appropriate modality with the client to address the presenting issue as well as any intersecting issues will apply. Naturally this will be the case whether one is a psychiatrist undertaking psychotherapy, a medical psychotherapist, a counselling psychologist, a clinical psychologist, or a psychotherapist. Given most readers will be entirely competent with such things, we will not needlessly detain ourselves here with a recap, but instead will move directly to a consideration of those matters which arise in psychotherapy which directly pertain to gender diverse people, before considering how gender diversity might be approached from the position of the more common psychotherapeutic modalities.

Coming Out

One of the key issues which many trans and non-binary people face is that of coming out, or telling others of their gender. People are often entirely sure that others will not be accepting. As ever in psychotherapy, when a client is entirely sure to the point of being unwilling to consider alternatives (if they say "Of course … " or "Everyone … " or some other such hyperbole), then right there is likely a part of the therapeutic puzzle – beneath that rigidity may very well be the change the client is unable to find themselves and has brought them to therapy. Happily, the general public in the United Kingdom and many other Western countries is often a good deal less interested in others being trans than is 'known' [feared] by the patient. Occasional bigotry aside, this tends to vary according to social distance from the client – people on the street are often uninterested, but partners or parents can be more so. An interesting exception is children who tend to be very accommodating – seeing it as simply another thing in a broadly incomprehensible world they are still learning about. The exception to *this* is where a partner endeavours to make the children less accommodating as a means of attack against the trans person.

---

[1] In the case of gender diversity, this would be use of the correct name and pronouns, ensuring toilet facilities are accommodating, and ensuring forms allow the person you are seeing to fill them in appropriately, for example.

This is an important point; people will very often claim that they themselves are accepting, but someone else will not be – whether that claim is made by a trans person who has reservations about coming out or another person who wishes the trans person to remain closeted. It is claimed that a child will not be accepting (they usually are) or an elderly person should not be told simply because they are old. This is rather ageist as older people tend to take a rather broader view, especially with those who are close to them – the argument that "they didn't have it in their day" being false (see Chapter 1, *Introduction*). All this is, in psychotherapeutic parlance, a form of displacement. It is easy to blame someone else; it means one doesn't have to take responsibility for one's own choices and feelings – the psychotherapeutic job here can be to leave these people outside of the therapy room and to attend to the feelings of the people actually present before moving on to speculations about others.

Similarly, a trans person simply stating that they will not tell a significant other about their gender may be viable if that person is never to be seen again; however, if they will be seen when ill, at a wedding, at a religious festival, or the like, then realistically some plan will need to be made, and not thinking about it is displacement from the presenting difficulty. Of course, in some cases there may be a real risk of violence and this will need to form part of the therapeutic consideration. As ever, gently getting details can pay dividends – the "violent and abusive" father could possibly be – and so thought, risk assessment and protection processes may need to be considered. However, it may be that their father has never actually been violent and indeed upon pressing is thought unlikely to be. Specificity is everything as it directs therapeutic action and attention.

Reality and Theory

Needless to say, both clients and clinicians should be wary of assumption – and certainly there will inevitably be problems. There are sometimes problems with living as a gender diverse person, but these are often related to intersections of marginalisation – to being trans and having a disability, for example, rather than to being trans per se. Consequently, safety behaviours such as clients *only* feeling able to access 'safe spaces' such as LGBT venues and *only* having LGBT friends may be usefully questioned. Of course, one may very well prefer these options – but that is very much not the same as feeling that they are the *only* possibilities. Indeed, it can be the case that some LGBT people are less accepting of gender diversity than some cisgender and heterosexual people because LGBT people have more skin in the game so to speak. For example, a gay man who has struggled with femininity may have more to say on the matter than someone who has not really thought about their gender.

In thinking about assumptions, we should also caution clinicians not to cleave too strongly to their modality's theory or writing on gender diversity from that theoretical standpoint.[2] Most modalities were developed in the past century, and in the case of psychodynamic approaches in fin-de-siècle Vienna. Gender has very much moved on from the ideas prevalent in those times and to use those ideas in a contemporary context would be as wrong as using medical techniques from that period. We may, of course, consider how gender might be approached from first principles within the modality and thus excise many of the cultural malignancies which have accrued; indeed, some principles

---

[2] Psychotherapeutic modalities can be a little like cults – with adherents, reified names who may not be questioned and are cited as "X tells us . . . ", and shouts of heresy when they are questioned. We suggest a rather more pragmatic approach which endeavours a dispassionate evaluation.

in this vein are outlined later in this chapter. The only exception to this may be psycho-dynamic approaches which are predicated upon what we now know to be a fallacious understanding of human gender and sexuality and so should generally not be used with this population.

This admonition to avoid assumption or over-theorisation also applies to other theoretical approaches such as queer theory, post-structuralism, or postmodernism to name but a few. These ideas have much to add to ideas of gender, but clients live in the real world where people study and work, pay bills, watch TV, and poke their 'phones. To deconstruct semiotics or to question whether the signifier is directly linked to the signified is all very well; ultimately, however, you need to have a name on your name badge or you are not going to get money from your job to buy bread and milk.

'Anxiety and Depression'

There is a sort of general malaise among some gender diverse people which is also covered in Chapter 4, *Mental Health Conditions*. It is a sort of low mood and anxiety, generally at just within clinical levels. It is often accompanied by a sometimes marked degree of social anxiety and does not seem to respond especially well to psychopharmacology, although for patients this is often the treatment of choice. It generally occurs around age 16 or so – essentially when the person is taking their first tentative steps into adulthood, and some of the parental and societal 'training wheels' are being removed. In its most severe incarnation, it resembles the [Japanese] phenomenon of hikikomori (Tamaki, 2013), with people spending their time in their childhood bedroom often playing computer games and with little [offline] social contact. Their parents usually support them financially and emotionally. In general, this phenomenon is caused by low self-esteem and a patient's feeling that the expectations placed upon them by modern society (whether the high degree of those demands or the lack of opportunity) are unrealisable. Consequently, psychopharmacology is of little effect, and shaming the person for their behaviours only worsens the problem (although naturally facilitating the situation is also damaging).

This phenomenon is not peculiar to gender diverse people – it is comparatively endemic in high-income technologically developed countries – however, it seems that in some cases fear of opprobrium for gender diversity can be a route in for those with a predisposition towards it. And perhaps in other cases, gender diversity can seem something of an excuse for social inhibition in a person where there was no previous gender dysphoria and no real-world testing to see if the gender suits.

It has been suggested that physical treatments such as hormones or surgeries will enable the person to leave their bedroom – an idea which can be enthusiastically received by the person's parents as both a reason and a 'cure' for their malaise and lethargy. It is not. Almost invariably the person simply stays where they were, only now even more concerned about fitting in with the wider world due to the physical changes effected in the absence of real-world testing.

A useful treatment can be a gentle graduated exposure to wider society (see *Cognitive Behavioural Therapy* in this chapter), with a simultaneous gentle withdrawal of the support mechanisms which allow the person to reside very comfortably at home. This may require caregivers to give up their parental roles, with all of the disquiet individuation always provokes. It can be uncomfortable, having been the person who gets to make the decisions, to have someone else making decisions – especially if they are ones you don't like. Clinicians can sometimes be co-opted into this power dynamic to ally with the caregiver in a "We're the adults aren't we?" way against the [adult] 'child' client – however, this must be avoided as this toxic relationship style may be at least partly to blame for the problem which has brought the client to therapy.

Graduated exposure may need to be very gradual indeed, and it can be good to start with something which is so simple as to seem almost silly – to go to the end of the garden path, for example. Most people will suggest that is too easy, but it will give a win upon which more challenging elements can be built. For those clients unwilling to do even the most simple of tasks, there may be useful therapeutic work in exploring why they will not engage in therapy in this way, and why they are so determined to articulate their distress through not engaging.

Sadly, a precipitating factor in social withdrawal can be school bullying, which is all too common among gender diverse people who, even if they were not out, were often gender atypical at that time. Here it is useful to identify safety behaviours which were developed by the child in response to the untenable situation they found themselves in – very commonly being trapped in an institution with one or more people who wished them harm. Behaviours such as avoidance are not unreasonable under such circumstances – however, they may be unconsciously applied by an adult in an adult situation where they have very many more options – without considering whether such tactics are still necessary or appropriate. Bringing all this to conscious awareness in the therapy room can allow the client to decide now, as an adult and given their current circumstances, what they wish to keep and what is best left in childhood.

Relationship Therapy

Relationships and sexuality are considered in some detail in Chapter 8, *Sexuality, Relationships, and Reproduction,* and will not be unnecessarily repeated here. Suffice to say that whatever one's modality, it is vital to be accepting of the wide variety of family and relationship forms, including consensual non-monogamy, monogamy, marriage, civil partnerships, personal arrangements, framily, and so on. Accommodation and adaptation may need to be made to usual procedures to accommodate these varieties of relationships, but this should not be insurmountable.

It is also vital not to situate a relationship problem in the client. As there is nothing inherently wrong with gender diversity, and as people have a wide variety of responses to it from the positive to the negative, there is no inevitable response – which means everyone is responsible for their reactions and will need to own them in the therapeutic space. Assertions of "Of course I can't live with a trans person" may be gently challenged, as should "Of course my wife would not be accepting" and so on. It may be that these issues are indeed the case at that time and for that client, but there is no "Of course" about it because this is not always the case (and indeed the veracity in this case may often be profitably investigated – has the conversation actually been had or is it supposition?). In the variability of possible responses is the room for therapeutic change. Further, not only is there therapeutic work to be done with the trans person and their significant others (who may also be trans, of course), but the relationship between them may also need addressing. Usually a sequential process involving each party in turn, and then all together, is valuable.

In contracting the therapeutic space to begin such work, ground rules may need to be agreed upon that things will be spoken about openly, about managing expressed emotion, about honesty, and possibly about name use, although this latter may better be grist for the therapeutic mill.

Groups

Group therapy for trans people is discussed in Richards (2014) largely from an existential perspective, although pluralistic principles are also outlined there and will be discussed later. One of the key benefits of groups in trans work is that they are excellent at challenging assumptions – one group member may hold something as being absolutely fundamentally true, for example, that one cannot be female without genital surgery; another may feel genital surgery is neither here nor there on the grounds that one's genitals are not on public display; and another may say it is hormones which are important as they affect how you feel; and so on. In each group member seeing the variety of opinions in the group, flexibility and change may be fostered.

Creating the opportunity for useful discussion can be challenging, and group facilitators may need to establish the group in such a way that it can best flourish. A first stage is to select group members who will be able to contribute and who will be neither too inhibited to contribute at all nor so narcissistic as to take the group over entirely.[3] Usually an open group is pragmatic as more members can be added as old ones leave; the interpersonal dynamics created by a closed group which are so important as a means of addressing some mental illnesses and complex trauma are not nearly so helpful in trans-specific work. Somewhere between 8–10 members for 1–1.5 hours seems to work well, with groups held either monthly or fortnightly for a year. This allows work to be done between times. Indeed, with gender diversity this work outside of the group is often fairly substantial, including coming out, telling people, investigating physical treatments, and so on. Consequently, a reasonable time elapsing between sessions facilitates this. As a happy side effect, it also allows people to travel further afield, meaning more people, or a wider variety of people, are able to participate.

Two group facilitators are useful, at least one of whom must be familiar with work with gender diverse people; both must be trained in group facilitation. The usual therapeutic practice will need to be adapted, and more intervention than usual may be necessary to keep things on track and spiralling up rather than down, as it were. This latter is important as groups can devolve into a discussion about how things are so bad, without thinking about meanings and solutions. This may be a reasonable start in a very long-term group; however, in most time-limited settings guidance from facilitators away from simple negativity and towards understanding and change will mean group members gain more from attendance during the sessions available.

Further to this, education may be needed about factual matters which then allows time for discussion. For example, a discussion about whether or not trans men can become pregnant on testosterone may be curtailed with the information that there is a chance, but it is not guaranteed; then an invitation to discuss what that means – what would barrier contraception methods mean? What would it mean to store gametes before physical treatments? What forms of sexual contact would feel good? And so on. Of course, this information could have been obtained over the progress of weeks; and there may have been useful digressions which have now been missed – but in general

---

[3] Remember we are considering groups specifically pertaining to gender diversity here. Groups which are not focused on gender may be just the place to address issues in communicating such as these.

when groups are judiciously managed in this way, it is unproductive talk which is avoided and productive discussion which is facilitated. Indeed, this principle of education on facts, then discussion of their impact and meaning, applies to relationship therapy and individual therapy also.

Reflexivity

In any therapeutic method or modality, being aware of oneself is vital, as it allows us to more accurately determine what in the room is down to us, what to the client, and what to the relationship. As suggested in the JoHari window, we need to try to reduce our unknown unknowns (Luft & Ingham, 1955); when working in gender diversity, it is naturally gender which forms the greater part of this introspection. For cisgender clinicians, it might be thought that there is not much to be known, as one's gender feels 'natural'; however, of course, it is not. Go back 100 years and it likely would have been expressed very differently. Go to any of a 100 different cultures globally and again it would be expressed differently; doubtless 100 years in the future it will be different again. It is simply that gender here and now has been learned from the very cradle and, due to meshing tightly with one's biology, feels simply right. Naturally, anything which is unconsidered is inimical to reflexivity; only by considering it both as something one is and something one does – and that one might possibly do something else – are we able to consider who we are and what we are doing at the moment. For this reason, cisgender people will have more work on gender reflexivity to do than trans people who have necessarily considered their gender already.

Trans clinicians too, however, will need to undertake gender reflexivity, not least because their gender will inevitably be different from that of their client even if they are from the same demographic background. For example, two 40-year-old trans women will have very different experiences of gender if one transitioned at age 10 and the other at age 39. Trans clinicians thinking of moving into gender work should also reflexively consider whether they have really dealt with their own gender issues because working in the same field as such a major upheaval in one's own life can act as a trigger which can spill over onto the client. You may find yourself desperate for a client to come to the same conclusion as you in what was apparently the same situation or indeed to make a different decision given the outcome you experienced. The insight and empathy of being the 'same' must be balanced against difference, and especially against whether potentially triggering situations can roll off you due to having being dealt with sufficiently in the past. Of course, this is not to say that only cisgender people may see trans people clinically, as many cisgender people are far from dispassionate about gender and may hold strong and unconsidered views they are almost unaware of and would also need addressing; it is simply that the same triggers may not apply.

Naturally all this is not peculiar to gender work – people in any field of clinical endeavour should consider well whether the drive and potential insight of being from approximately the same demographic as one's clients is adequately balanced against potentially having investment in the client's outcomes for reasons other than the best interest of the client. This may profitably be considered when alone, perhaps in a park or coffee shop, or in personal therapy or supervision. There is no right answer, except to be honest and to honestly consider the issue.

Person-centred Therapy

Person-centred therapy can be of great use to trans clients in that it allows space to explore and is generally methodologically accepting of diversity. This space must be an active space – simply sitting quietly won't do. Silence can be open and accepting or passive aggressive, and/or lazy. As with any therapeutic intervention, it must be used judiciously, deliberately, and not overmuch.[4]

The unconditional positive regard which is a mainstay of this modality can create a useful opportunity for people to test out identities or to feel acceptance when others are negatively judging. This can be a useful place for some clients to explore feelings of shame, especially if it is shame which has been encultured from childhood or has been reinforced through adult relationships and so feels intractable in everyday life.

There is also a place for *congruence* in the sense meant within person-centred therapy; however, clinicians unfamiliar with gender diversity may find that they are experiencing reactions to the person's gender which are far more about themselves than their client or their relationship with the client. For this reason, the steps taken in relation to reflexivity noted earlier are vital, and clinicians unfamiliar with the field should use interventions based on congruence extremely carefully.

Psychodynamic Approaches.

Psychodynamic approaches, whether psychoanalysis, psychodynamic psychotherapy, or to a lesser extent cognitive analytic therapy and its variations, are not useful for working with trans and non-binary people: At base, these approaches take a stance which is inimical to gender diversity in that they assume a binary model of gender with a heterocentric cisgender norm and consider variation from that to be deviant. While some workers have endeavoured to formulate a more inclusive stance, this necessarily has to eschew a great body of work by many of the founders and luminaries in the field who were cissexist and heterosexist (indeed at times actively transphobic and homophobic) and so creates inherent tensions which are inevitably played out in the therapist, the client, and the relationship.

The old theorising of [binary] trans identities being caused by over-identification with the 'opposite' sex parent are fallacious (leaving aside the assumption of heterosexual parents in a relationship). This is a re-heating of the suggestion that same-sex attraction is caused by over-identification with the 'opposite sex' parent. It was proven incorrect for same-sex attraction and also for trans people (Zucker, 2008). Indeed a moment's thought shows that it will not be so. Consider the number of boys raised by mothers where the father is absent (and therefore the boy may only identify with the mother as parent) – we should expect vastly more trans girls than trans boys therefore, and yet this is not the case, with numbers being slightly reversed.

Sadly this unfounded theorisation has had negative real-world effects with children removed from trans parents on the flawed psychodynamic theorisation that trans people are necessarily unfit parents. Of course, being trans does not make one an unfit parent. Sadly

---

[4] Do note that the tired sophistry about client anxiety with silence being part of the therapy is *almost* always just a means of the therapist abrogating responsibility for the outcome of the therapy onto the client. Taken to reducto ad absurdum, the same argument would apply if you simply didn't turn up for the session and left them to manage their anxiety while you read a book in a coffee shop with a slice of cake.

this echoes past damage caused by psychodynamic theorisation including the incorrect assertion that same-sex partnered people could not be appropriate parents, autism being caused by 'cold and distant mothers' (and again children being removed from their parents), and the absurd 'schizophrenogenic mother'. In general, therefore, another modality is best with this client group.

Cognitive Behavioural Therapy (CBT)

CBT[5] is a very common evidence-based therapeutic modality which has no especial axiomatic view on gender diversity, and which may usefully be employed in the service of gender diverse people who are experiencing difficulties. Indeed, being a cognitive *behavioural* therapy, it is especially well placed to aid in testing out negative assumptions in the real world through graduated exposure. For example, if someone who was assigned male at birth is concerned about wearing a skirt in public, then they can try doing so in a safe environment (perhaps alone in a bedroom), before widening out to trusted friends, and then outside, before work or parents and so on – with each stage building upon the last – just as one would with a general client who has a phobic reaction to using public transport, for example.

Similarly the usual interventions one would use to address the developed schema and negative automatic thoughts derived from problematic childhood experiences can profitably be employed in gender work. The identification of "Of course . . . " and "Obviously . . . " statements and the cognitions and indeed feelings which occur in response to gender-related circumstances or stimuli can be unpacked and new ideas brought into awareness and tried out.

The idea that being trans or non-binary is Not OK can be very deeply embedded and may take considerable work to undo, but the effort is worthwhile as the change can be remarkable. Indeed this is one of the few cases where the therapist's own professional standing can usefully be employed to counteract negative messages which have been received. The client may have had a teacher who told them they were foolish for wanting to wear a skirt from the dress-up box as a child and internalised the idea that authority is not accepting of that wish. For a consultant psychiatrist or consultant psychologist to say otherwise – not to be neutral but to actively say that it is entirely reasonable – can counteract that negative message extremely effectively.[6] Note that this is not telling the client to wear a skirt, simply that it is absolutely fine if they wish to. Finally, it has to be absolutely fine – not fine if they can't help it or fine because they were made that way. Simply that the act in and of itself is harmless and therefore fundamentally OK.

Another area CBT can be of assistance is, of course, that of cognitions; here again usual practice may be adapted. For example, if a client is catastrophising about not being 'safe' going out due to fear of attack, the evidence can be considered. Specific questioning

---

[5] In a book which considers gender and sexuality, we should note that one really *must* be able to competently differentiate this from other uses of the same acronym.

[6] This point about neutrality is an important general principle. While we must hold open the possibility for a client to interpret their own world, a neutral response to an egregious wrong such as the murder of a child, for example, is not 'neutral' in any human sense. In some instances, a neutral response becomes a valanced response (in this case, more positive than one would expect) due to the normative human response being of a very different valance. While the therapeutic modality is vital, so too is recognising that there are two humans in the room.

can be useful as "Everyone gets jumped on and murdered" could change to "I always get attacked when I go out" to "I haven't been attacked as such, but my friend has, and I've been abused by people" to "I read about a person online being attacked and I think the people were laughing at me." Of course some trans people do get attacked, but it is happily rarer than often feared (although higher than for the cisgender population in some contexts). However, there is a salience effect wherein people who are abused tell others, whereas people who have had quotidian days do not. It's similar to plane crashes, which do occur, but where only crashes rather than successful flights are reported, and so those tragedies are much more prominent and thus unduly influence those who are prone to such influence – especially if that reporting was all the exposure they have had to the phenomenon.

Existentialism

The existential approaches are usually accepting of diversity – predicated as they are on a search for meaning and authenticity, and being shot through with a distaste for accepted societal dogma. The axiomatic point of contention is over the existential Givens – those things considered to be immutable to human Being, defined as death, freedom, isolation, and meaning. As many people also consider their gender and sexuality to be an immutable part of who they are, they therefore find the idea that these may be ephemeral to be wrong and (when voiced by people with the privilege of a normative gender or sexuality and who therefore have implicit identities which accord with their own understandings) offensive. The philosophy behind this need not trouble us here but is exhaustively explored in Richards (2017). Suffice to say that where theoretical considerations come into conflict with real people's lives, the ethics and ethical treatment of people must take precedence (Richards, 2017).

Givens aside, several useful concepts from existential therapy may be employed with trans clients. The first of these is the notion of existential authenticity – that is, being oneself and so being eudemonic: in being able to be oneself, one is more content (happiness is too slippery a concept to aim for). Of course, we are born into a world which already exists and has certain restrictions, so we cannot entirely be ourselves, as we must live with others where ourselves may impinge on theirselves, causing them to impinge on us and so on. However, that is the nature of being in a world with others and negotiating that is the task of humans. Naturally, the therapeutic endeavour may be about exploring the specifics of what gender one is (one's authenticity) and how that may be realised in the world (being in the world with others).

In living authentically, one is more able to pursue one's *project* – the thing which gives one's life meaning and purpose whatever those may be. For some trans people, it may be the process of transition, but this can be a little hollow after a while – it is almost as if gender is what one lives *through* or *as* rather than what one lives *for*. The client who says that they are not working, studying, or socialising because they are "doing this" (i.e. transitioning) never seems to be doing especially much or especially well.

The existential point of being-with-others is important, as isolation is far more likely if one is not able to relate to others as oneself. Many trans people report that while they had many friends pre-transition, they felt lonely and isolated as "no one really knew me"; indeed, when someone did get close, they only got so close before a barrier in relating appeared – whereas after transition they felt much more relaxed and able to connect with others.

The decision to transition is often bounded by the freedom the person has. Within the existential canon, freedom is important because it is often far greater than the person wishes to contemplate[7] but carries with it the burden of responsibility for the choices one has made within that freedom. Within gender therapy, identifying the edges of what are assumptions and what are concrete realities of the world can be extremely illuminating; here, perhaps more than anywhere, the therapist will need to be reflexively aware of their own assumptions and biases around gender. The use of open horizontalisation (with no therapist interpretation) to explore ideas which may appear unrelated but which may be, can be invaluable.

Some people who are exploring ideas around gender can make decisions such as to transition in a timely manner (those who choose); some can carry on as usual asserting they have no freedom – which is almost never the case, although the cost may be great (those who choose not to choose); and some come to therapy, or gender clinics, or read about gender and talk for year after year after year but do not act to explore beyond this (those who choose to keep choosing). In all cases, bringing into awareness what the person is doing and considering if they want to do it (and in that way) are useful interventions.

In deciding whether or not to transition, it is not uncommon for some people whose disposition is inclined that way to wish to have things organised such that there is no possibility of error before making the final step of coming out. Naturally good organisation can avoid unwanted and unexpected problems; however, with some trans people the organisation can be pathological in that it acts as a safety behaviour which prevents the person from actually acting, as it assuages just enough drive through planning but is never entirely satisfactory. It is like reading the menu and considering what one might eat in a restaurant – sensible to a point, but after too long perhaps it hides an underlying reluctance. Existentially, the notion of a leap-to-faith is important to address this. Note it is correctly a leap *to* faith, not the popularly bowdlerised leap of faith. The idea (from Kierkegaard, 1980 [1844]) is that one cannot move from a position of logical certainty to a position of [religious] faith through a series of intermediate steps – one must make a *leap* from one to the other. For our purposes here, there is ultimately no interim step between being closeted and being out about one's gender. One can prepare, but at some point one must screw one's courage to the sticking point and actually *tell* someone. Of course, this is the same with many things in life – the first kiss, the job interview, the slap for the final hold on the rock wall – you do or you don't.

Lastly, and perhaps appositely, comes death, and the movement towards it – finitude. This is the idea that at some point we all must die; we will have forged the sum total of our deeds – for good or ill – and must accept that as our lot. In considering this, many trans people understandably wish to ensure that they have lived as themselves, at least for a little while. Indeed, some trans people nearing death wish to be buried as themselves. As ageing progresses, some trans people take stock once again of the things they felt prohibited them from transitioning: are any children grown; have they retired from the job; have their spouse or parents passed on? (See Chapter 8, *Sexuality, Relationships, and Reproduction*.) There can be regret that they had not transitioned earlier or a feeling that it is now too late – but there are, of course, losses and gains to each.[8] Very often, people imagine that had they

---

[7] To the point of nausea indeed.

[8] There is no absolute upper limit. Certainly we have seen people in their 90s in gender identity clinics. As with any other medical treatment, physical treatments are predicated on health, rather than age.

transitioned earlier in life, they would have had the life they have experienced, but in a different gender – when of course that would not have been the case. At the very least, it is unlikely that they would have had the precise children they had if they had transitioned early on. A sensible exploration of what life might actually have been like, and what it still could be like, can be both healing and hopeful.

Summary

In summary, for most therapeutic approaches, the usual modes of intervention can be used while adapting them for trans and non-binary clients. While specialised therapy may be needed on some occasions – if there are complex interactions with hormones, surgeries, or sex offending, for example – in general a qualified therapist should be able to manage therapy for trans and non-binary people entirely competently. The only caveat is that if one is to mix modalities, one must be familiar with them so as to avoid tripping up on the fractures between them. For example, if one wishes to use both existential and CBT approaches, one must be able to manage the differing understandings of awareness and anxiety between them. If that can be done competently, the only common tripping point is an overemphasis on the client's trans status, and ignoring, or underemphasising the very many other aspects which inevitably make up the complex human before you.

Further Reading

Beattie, M., & Lenihan, P. (2018). *Counselling skills for working with gender diversity and identity*. London: Jessica Kingsley Publishers.

Lev, A. I. (2004). *Transgender emergence*. London: Haworth Clinical Practice Press.

Richards, C. (2011). Transsexualism and existentialism. *Existential Analysis, 22* (2), 272–279.

(2014). Trans and existentialism. In M. Milton (ed.). *Sexuality: Existential perspectives* (pp. 217–230). Ross-on-Wye: PCCS Books.

Richards, C., & Barker. M. (2013). *Sexuality and gender for mental health professionals: A practical guide*. London: Sage.

References

Kierkegaard, S. (1980 [1844]). *The concept of anxiety* [trans R. Thomte and

A. B. Anderson]. Princeton, NJ: Princeton University Press.

Luft, J., & Ingham, H. (1955). The Johari window: A graphic model of interpersonal awareness. In J. Luft (1969), *Of human interaction* (p. 177). Palo Alto, CA: National Press.

(2014). Group therapy and sexuality. In M. Milton (ed.). *Sexuality: Existential perspectives* (pp. 265–284). Ross-on-Wye: PCCS Books.

Richards, C. (2017). [Monograph]. *Trans and sexuality: An existentially-informed ethical enquiry with implications for counselling psychology*. London: Routledge.

Tamaki, S. (2013). *Hikikomori: Adolescence without end*. Minneapolis: University of Minnesota Press.

Zucker, K. (2008). Children with gender identity disorder: Is there a best practice? *Neuropsychiatrie de l'enfance et de l'adolescence 56*, 358–364.

Index

abdominal aortic aneurysm,
    screening for, 38
abuse
    dealing with in school, 28
    of gender atypical
        children, 14
    terms of, 9
age
    and change of name, 94
    and hormone therapy, 37
    of majority in the UK, 6
    and testosterone levels, 32
agender people
    definition, 2
Albert Kennedy Trust (www
    .akt.org.uk), 93
alcohol, 26, 40
amateur dramatic societies,
    and trans people with
    ASC, 77
androphile, 81
anorexia, 15
anti-epileptic medication, 40
anxiety
    diagnosis in trans
        people, 46
    evolution of humans to
        notice, 75
    graded exposure to, 72
    marginalisation stress
        and, 55
    prejudice and, 45
    psychotherapy, 108-9
appearance, help with for trans
    people with ASC, 77-9
asexuality, 86
Asperger's syndrome, 70
assessment
    adaptations, 15
    asking about hormones or
        surgeries, 16
    forms of, 14
    general assessment of trans
        people, 15-17
    for hormones and surgeries.
        see specialist assessment
    rapport and, 15
    respecting gender as
        requirement of, 15

summary, 29
    use of preferred name and
        pronouns, 15
assigned at birth, use of the
    term, 4
*assigned female at birth
    (AFAB)*, 4
*assigned male at birth
    (AMAB)*, 4
augmentation
    mammoplasty, 42
autism, 70, 113
autistic spectrum
    conditions (ASC)
    association with cosplay and
        gender dysphoria,
        10-11
    Brony identification and, 12
    childhood
        presentations, 71-2
    and confusion of traits,
        70, 71
    and diagnosis, 72
    discrimination, 79
    gender dysphoria and,
        71-2, 73
    help with appearance, 77-9
    institutional responses, 75
    making new friends as
        a trans person
        with, 75-7
    prevalence in the general
        population, 70
    prevalence in trans
        people, 46
    sexuality, 72-3
    and specialist assessment, 20
    and treatment, 72 *see also*
        intellectual
        disability (ID)
aversion treatment, 17, 54

Barker, M., 37, 82, 116
BDSM (Bondage and
    Discipline, Dominance
    and Submission, and
    Sadomasochism), 10,
    81, 82-3
Bellringer, J., 42

binary trans people,
    definition, 2
binder, 6, 41
bipolar disorder, 48
birth certificates, 95, 97
blood tests, 37
body dysmorphic disorder
    (BDD), 19
    and gender dysphoria, 19, 51
    as mental health
        condition, 50-1
body fat, 32, 35
body hair, 35
body mass index (BMI), 27, 34,
    37, 42, 43
body parts, examples of
    language used by trans
    people, 85-6
borderline personality
    disorder, 49-50
Bouman, W. P., 116
bowel cancer, screening for, 38
breast cancer, 37, 39, 85
    screening for, 38
breast implants, 38
British Association for Sexual
    Health and HIV
    (BASHH), 2, 87
British Association of Gender
    Identity Specialists
    (BAGIS), 5, 17
British Psychological Society
    (BPS), 54
British Psychological Society's
    *Guidelines for assessment,
    formulation, and
    diagnosis* (BPS,
    forthcoming 2021), 17
Bronies, 11-12
Buddhism, view of sexual
    orientation and gender
    identity, 104
bullying, 28, 64, 88, 109

cachet, of being trans, 20
Cancer Research UK, 37
cannabis, 40
categorisations, for trans and
    non-binary people, 2-3